# Essentials of Card  thesia

# Essentials of Cardiac and Thoracic Anaesthesia

**John W. W. Gothard** FRCA

**Andrea Kelleher** FRCA

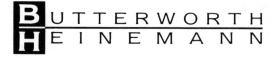

OXFORD   AUCKLAND   BOSTON   JOHANNESBURG   MELBOURNE   NEW DELHI

Butterworth-Heinemann
Linacre House, Jordan Hill, Oxford OX2 8DP
225 Wildwood Avenue, Woburn, MA 01801-2041
A division of Reed Educational and Professional Publishing Ltd

℞ A member of the Reed Elsevier plc group

First published 1999
Reprinted 2000

**British Library Cataloguing in Publication Data**
A catalogue record for this book is available from the British Library

**Library of Congress Cataloguing in Publication Data**
A catalogue record for this book is avialable from the Library of Congress

ISBN 0 7506 2033 1

Typeset by Genesis Typesetting, Rochester, kent
Printed and bound in Great Britain by Biddles Ltd, *www.Biddles.co.uk*

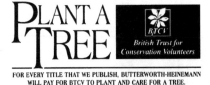

# Contents

# Preface

Changes in the training of anaesthetists has prompted us to produce this new textbook, *Essentials of Cardiac and Thoracic Anaesthesia*. Specialist registrars in anaesthesia are likely to be less experienced when they first meet the problems of cardiothoracic anaesthesia in the future. This book is intended therefore as a guide to this group of anaesthetists. It is hoped, however, that *Essentials of Cardiac and Thoracic Anaesthesia* will also be of interest to specialist nurses and anaesthetic technicians working in intensive care and in the operating theatre.

The book covers, in separate sections, both cardiac and thoracic anaesthesia. The reader is taken through the basic anaesthetic sequence of pre-operative assessment, intra-operative management and postoperative care for both forms of surgery in the adult. The information is presented in a straightforward manner and is intended as a practical guide to cardiothoracic anaesthesia. The text is not profusely referenced as the book is intended to be didactic rather than discoursive. Appropriate references are included, however, to justify more controversial areas of practice and also to illustrate the development of cardiothoracic anaesthesia.

We are grateful to both anaesthetic and surgical colleagues at the Royal Brompton Hospital for advice in the preparation of this book. Finally, we would like to express sincere thanks to our families, who have supported us throughout the project.

*John W. W. Gothard*
*Andrea Kelleher*

# Chapter 1

# Pre-operative assessment – cardiac anaesthesia

## Introduction

The anaesthetic assessment of the patient presenting for cardiac surgery is, potentially, a time-consuming and yet essential task. This assessment should, preferably, be undertaken by an anaesthetist who will be involved in the intra-operative care of the patient. In a busy cardiac surgical unit the anaesthetist making the pre-operative visit has, in practice, to make a fairly rapid assessment of the patient on the basis of a medical history which has already been elucidated, and on the results of general medical and specific cardiological investigations available in the case notes. In specific circumstances individual aspects of the patient's pre-operative condition will merit further questioning and examination of the patient. In addition, further investigations may be required before surgery is undertaken.

The pre-operative visit also provides the anaesthetist with an opportunity to explain to the patient how anaesthesia will be conducted. This should include an explanation of premedication, induction of anaesthesia (including the siting of invasive monitoring lines under local anaesthesia) and the possibility of elective mechanical ventilation postoperatively. Much of this detail may have been discussed with the patient previously by the nursing and physiotherapy staff, or possibly explained in an introductory programme. An informed explanation of future events by the anaesthetist to be involved in the case remains advisable and is essential in the high-risk case.

The following discussion of pre-operative assessment is divided into several sections for the sake of clarity. Many of the sections overlap to some extent and cannot be put in firm chronological order. For example, the management of drug therapy is discussed separately but will also need to be considered in the general anaesthetic assessment of the patient. Tables 1.1–1.12 summarize the important features of the pre-operative assessment.

## General anaesthetic assessment

The cardiological and surgical aspects of the cardiac patient will have been fully investigated and evaluated prior to surgery by the appropriate medical and surgical teams. The relevance of other, non-cardiac, medical disease to the management of the patient in the peri-operative period must not, however, be overlooked. Furthermore other factors which are specifically relevant to anaesthesia often go unnoticed by non-anaesthetists (e.g. previous anaesthetic history, anatomic features predisposing to difficult endotracheal intubation, a recent chest infection or anaesthetic drug allergies). The general anaesthetic assessment is therefore of paramount importance. A proforma for the general anaesthetic assessment of the cardiac surgical patient combined with a brief summary of relevant cardiological and general investigations is detailed in Table 1.1.

The presence of concomitant medical disease may be purely coincidental in the cardiac surgical patient but some disease processes such as diabetes and hyperlipidaemia predispose to cardiac pathology and ischaemic heart disease in particular. Other risk factors for coronary artery disease (Table 1.2) are linked to pathology in other systems which will need to be assessed pre-operatively (e.g. smoking and lung function). Hypertension and cigarette smoking not only

**Table 1.1 Proforma for cardiac anaesthetic assessment**

| | | | | | |
|---|---|---|---|---|---|
| Name: | No: | Age: | Sex: | Wt: | (kg) |
| | | | | Ht: | (cm) |

Diagnosis:

Planned operation:

Other medical problems?

| Drugs: | 1. | 2. | 3. | 4. |
|---|---|---|---|---|
| | 5. | 6. | 7. | 8. |

*General anaesthetic questionnaire*

Previous anaesthetics:

Allergies:

| | | |
|---|---|---|
| GO reflux: | Mouth opening: | |
| Neck movement: | Teeth: | Grade of intubation: |

| Cardiovascular status: | | | |
|---|---|---|---|
| BP:    (mmHg) | Hypertension? | Heart failure? | MI? |

Echocardiography:

Angiography:

| | | |
|---|---|---|
| LVEDP:    (mmHg) | Ejection fraction:    (%) | |

| Respiratory status: | | |
|---|---|---|
| Smoking history? | COPD? | Asthma? |
| $FEV_1$/FVC: | PEFR: | $PaO_2$/$PaCO_2$ |
| Chest X-ray: | | |

| Results: | Urea: | Hb: | Blood cross-matched: | |
|---|---|---|---|---|
| | Creatinine: | Platelet count: | | |
| | Potassium: | Coag screen: | INR: | APTT: |

**Table 1.2 Risk factors for coronary artery disease**

---

Age
Sex (M>F)
Race
Increased blood lipids, particularly low density lipoprotein (LDL)
Hypertension
Cigarette smoking
Diabetes mellitus
Family history
Overweight and obesity
Sedentary existence

---

increase the risk of atheroma in the coronary arteries but are also implicated in the formation of atheroma elsewhere in the arterial tree. This has specific relevance to cardiac surgery for the following reasons:

*Carotid stenosis*
● Symptomatic carotid stenosis increases the risk of cerebral damage during cardiopulmonary bypass. Pre-operative carotid endarterectomy may be indicated. Internal carotid stenoses of 70% which are detected in the asymptomatic patient may also warrant surgical intervention prior to cardiac surgery.

*Atheroma of ascending aorta*
● Makes cross-clamping of the aorta difficult
● Possibility of dislodging plaque elsewhere into the circulation (NB cerebral and coronary vessels).

*Abdominal aortic aneurysm*
● Possibility of rupture
● Gut ischaemia (a rare but disastrous complication following cardiac surgery) more likely?

*Renal artery stenosis*
● Poor renal function. Renal failure more likely postoperatively.

*Iliac and femoral artery atheroma*
● Makes passage of an intra-aortic balloon pump difficult and hazardous.
● Femoral arterial cannulation difficult.

*Distal limb ischaemia*
● Poor skin healing when veins harvested for coronary surgery (particularly lower leg).

## Risk assessment

It is important for the patient to know the risk of the operation they are about to undergo in terms of mortality and morbidity. A knowledge of these risks for individual patients also aids the audit of surgical results and allows a rational use of hospital resources.

A simple scoring system such as the American Society of Anesthesiologists classification (ASA status) categorizes the disease state of the patient and the New York Heart Association functional classification of angina assesses cardiovascular disability of patients. The Canadian Classification of Effort Angina is another commonly used functional classification (Tables 1.3–1.5). Physical status alone is not, however, an absolute indicator of operative risk or morbidity. A number of scoring systems have therefore been developed specifically to predict the outcome of cardiac surgery on the basis of known pre-operative risk factors. These scoring systems can be used to estimate the probability of mortality after cardiac surgery but are less accurate in predicting

**Table 1.3 American Society of Anesthesiologists (ASA) classification of physical status**

| | |
|---|---|
| ASA 1 | The patient has no organic, physiological, biochemical or psychiatric disturbance. The pathological process for which operation is to be performed is localized and does not entail a systemic disturbance |
| ASA 2 | Mild to moderate systemic disturbance caused either by the condition to be treated surgically or by other pathophysiological processes. Examples are mild organic heart disease, diabetes, mild hypertension, anaemia, old age, obesity and mild chronic bronchitis |
| ASA 3 | Limitation of life-style. Severe systemic disturbance or disease from whatever cause, even though it may not be possible to define the degree of disability with any finality, e.g. angina, healed myocardial infarction, severe diabetes and cardiac failure |
| ASA 4 | Severe symptomatic disorders that are already life threatening, not always correctable by operation, e.g. marked cardiac insufficiency, persistent angina, active myocarditis, advanced pulmonary, renal, endocrine or hepatic insufficiency |
| ASA 5 | Moribund. Little chance of survival, but submitted to operation in desperation |
| | Note: If the operation is an emergency, the letter E is placed by the numerical classification, and the patient is considered to be in poorer physical condition |

**Table 1.4 New York Heart Association functional classification**

| | |
|---|---|
| Class I | Patients with cardiac disease but without resulting limitations of physical activity. Ordinary physical activity does not cause undue fatigue, palpitations, dyspnoea or anginal pain |
| Class II | Patients with cardiac disease resulting in slight limitation of physical activity. They are comfortable at rest. Ordinary physical activity results in fatigue, palpitations, dyspnoea or anginal pain |
| Class III | Patients with cardiac disease resulting in marked limitation of physical activity. They are comfortable at rest. Less than ordinary physical activity causes fatigue, palpitations, dyspnoea or anginal pain |
| Class IV | Patients with cardiac disease resulting in inability to carry on any physical activity without discomfort. Symptoms of cardiac insufficiency or of the anginal syndrome may be present even at rest. If any physical activity is undertaken discomfort is increased |

**Table 1.5 Canadian Cardiovascular Society classification of effort angina**

| | |
|---|---|
| Class I | Ordinary physical activity, such as walking and climbing stairs does not cause angina. Angina occurs with strenuous or rapid or prolonged exertion at work or recreation |
| Class II | Slight limitation of ordinary activity. Angina occurs with walking or climbing stairs rapidly, walking uphill, walking or stair climbing after meals, or in cold, or in wind, or under emotional stress, or only during the few hours after awakening. Angina occurs when walking more than two blocks on the level or climbing more than one flight of ordinary stairs at normal pace and in normal conditions |
| Class III | Marked limitation of ordinary physical activity. Angina occurs with walking one to two blocks on the level and climbing one flight of stairs in normal conditions and at a normal pace |
| Class IV | Inability to carry on any physical activity without discomfort – angina may be present at rest |

From Campeau (1975)

**Table 1.6 Parsonnet's risk scoring for adult cardiac surgery**

| Risk factor | Parsonnet score |
|---|---|
| **Female gender** | 1 |
| Morbid obesity (>1.5 × ideal weight) | 3 |
| Diabetes (unspecified type) | 3 |
| Hypertension (systolic >140 mmHg) | 3 |
| Ejection fraction (%) | |
| >50 | 0 |
| 30–49 | 2 |
| <30 | 4 |
| Age (years) | |
| 70–74 | 7 |
| 75–79 | 12 |
| >80 | 20 |
| Re-operation | |
| 1st | 5 |
| 2nd | 10 |
| Pre-operative IABP | 2 |
| LV aneurysm | 5 |
| Emergency surgery (e.g. from catheter laboratory) | 10 |
| Dialysis dependent | 10 |
| Catastrophic state (e.g. cardiogenic shock, acute renal failure) | 10–50 |
| Other factors (paced, asthma) | 2–10 |
| Valve surgery | |
| Mitral | 5 |
| PA pressure >60 mmHg | 8 |
| Aortic | 5 |
| Pressure gradient >120 mmHg | 7 |
| CABG at time of valve surgery | 2 |

IABP, intra-aortic balloon pump; LV, left ventricular; PA, pulmonary artery;
CABG, coronary bypass graft. From Parsonnet *et al.* (1989)

**Table 1.7 Use of Parsonnet score to predict risk of surgery**

| Parsonnet score | Risk | Mortality (%) |
|---|---|---|
| 0–4 | Good | 1 |
| 5–9 | Fair | 5 |
| 10–14 | Poor | 9 |
| 15–19 | High | 17 |
| 20+ | Extremely high | 30 |

From Parsonnet *et al.* (**1989**)

morbidity. The scores only determine the likelihood of mortality in a large number of patients and are not sensitive enough to predict the outcome for individual patients.

The scoring system developed by Victor Parsonnet, an American surgeon, is now widely used to predict mortality (Tables 1.6 and 1.7). This risk classification has, however, been criticized because it tends to overestimate mortality and is subjective for some of the scores such as 'catastrophic states'. A variety of other scoring methods are therefore in use including that of the Association of Cardiothoracic Anaesthetists of Great Britain (ACTA) and other systems involving Bayesian analysis of risk factors (Stedmon *et al.*, 1995). Finally, the Association of Thoracic Surgeons of Great Britain and Ireland produce annual mortality figures for cardiac surgery in the United Kingdom. These figures are produced somewhat in arrears and as an amalgamation do not reflect results in individual units (which should also be available annually). They are, however, useful in providing an overall view of mortality. The latest available figures are summarized in Table 1.8.

# Identification of 'fast-track' patients

Many units now try and identify low-risk patients who can be allowed to breathe spontaneously early in the postoperative period following cardiac surgery. It is often possible to remove the endotracheal tube within a few hours of surgery in this group of patients. Early 'extubation' in an uncomplicated patient who is not bleeding and is not requiring inotropic support has a number of advantages, particularly relating to the use of available resources. These patients can be managed outside the main intensive care unit, albeit initially in a high-

**Table 1.8 Mortality for cardiac surgery 1995–1996**

| | Numbers of procedures | Deaths (%) |
|---|---|---|
| CABG alone | 22 475 | 3.7 |
| Aortic valve only | 2724 | 4.4 |
| Mitral valve only | 1405 | 4.8 |
| CABG plus valve | 2085 | 7.6 |

UK Cardiac Surgical Register results from 38 of 40 NHS units

**Table 1.9 Selection criteria for 'fast-track' patients**

1. Age up to 74 years
2. Parsonnet score less than 10
3. Absence of significant lung disease or condition that may compromise postoperative respiratory function
4. Less than 30% overweight by standard body mass index
5. Hypertension, if present, must be controlled
6. Controlled blood glucose if diabetic
7. Left ventricular ejection fraction >30%, or >50% if myocardial infarction within last month
8. Surgery for:
     First time coronary artery bypass grafting (CABG)
     First time aortic valve surgery with or without CABG
     Simple congenital repair (e.g. ASD – no pulmonary hypertension)
     NB mitral valve surgery *not* included
9. Aspirin must have been stopped for 7 days pre-operatively (or platelets pre-ordered?)
10. No neurological deficit
11. Absence of other systemic condition that may compromise a rapid recovery from surgery

dependency area with full monitoring and ventilatory facilities. After extubation a stable patient may be transferred to a less intensive high-dependency area, or nursing care can be stepped down somewhat in the same area. This type of system (now designated by the unfortunate term 'fast-track' system in many hospitals) is claimed to cut the cost of uncomplicated cardiac surgery without compromising standards of care. It is also put forward that early extubation of low-risk patients could be beneficial and may lead to an earlier discharge from hospital. The possibility that silent ischaemia can occur in patients extubated very early in the postoperative period following coronary artery surgery has not yet been fully investigated, however.

The criteria for selection of 'fast-track' patients in our unit are listed in Table 1.9. The anaesthetic management of these patients is discussed further in Chapters 2 to 5.

# Investigations – relevance to cardiac surgery

## General investigations

All patients require a recent chest X-ray, a full blood count, blood sugar, urea and electrolyte measurements and blood coagulation studies. If not previously measured, liver function tests and a lipid profile should be requested. In addition, some clinicians would prefer to know the patient's hepatitis B antigen status and whether they are carriers of methicillin-resistant *Staphylococcus aureus* (MRSA). For most cardiac procedures 4 units of blood are cross-matched prior to surgery but for re-operations 6–8 units should be available. The interpretation of general investigations in respect of planned cardiac surgery is detailed in the following section.

## Chest X-ray

Postero-anterior (PA) and lateral films are taken routinely and reveal the size and shape of the heart, atria and great vessels, the degree of vascularization of the lung fields and the presence of aortic, valvar or pericardial calcification and pleural/pericardial effusions. The lateral film can also be used to estimate the proximity of the heart and great vessels to the back of the sternum in patients scheduled for re-operation. More detailed information on this latter point can be derived from computed tomographic (CT) scanning or nuclear magnetic resonance (NMR) techniques.

Abnormalities on the pre-operative chest X-ray may relate solely to existing cardiac disease, for example ventricular hypertrophy with aortic stenosis, pulmonary oedema in left ventricular failure or upper lobe blood diversion in patients with pulmonary venous hypertension (e.g. mitral stenosis). Abnormalities attributable to smoking-related lung disease, such as small bullae and emphysematous changes, may be present in patients scheduled for coronary artery surgery. These changes may forewarn of technical problems with internal mammary artery grafting, because of lung distension, or possible difficulty with weaning from mechanical ventilation. Occasionally an asymptomatic carcinoma of the bronchus is detected. Finally, the pre-operative chest X-ray will inevitably provide an invaluable baseline with which to compare postoperative chest X-rays.

## Abnormalities of other routine tests

### Full blood count

#### Anaemia
A haemoglobin of less than 10 g/dl will lead to excessive haemodilution during cardiopulmonary bypass, particularly in small patients. Transfusion will almost certainly be necessary, although haemofiltration may be an alternative option. The aetiology of the anaemia may be relevant to management. For example, dietary iron deficiency anaemia, thalassaemia minor and the anaemia of sickle cell trait can be managed with blood transfusion. Evidence of bleeding from a duodenal ulcer, hiatus hernia or colonic carcinoma is much more serious because any bleeding tendency will be exacerbated on bypass due to full heparinization. In addition postoperative gastrointestinal haemorrhage requiring surgical intervention carries a mortality of approximately 50% following cardiac surgery.

#### Thrombocytopenia
Platelet function is abnormal after cardiopulmonary bypass and in patients treated with aspirin and other anti-platelet agents. A low platelet count will increase the likelihood of postoperative bleeding. The aetiology of the low count should be investigated if time allows but in any case platelet concentrate should be available for transfusion in the postoperative period. The management of aspirin and anti-coagulant drug therapy in the peri-operative period is discussed later in this chapter.

### Clotting studies

Abnormal clotting studies in the cardiac surgical patient are commonly due to:

*Drug therapy*
Aspirin/dipyrimadole (platelet inhibition)
Non-steroidal anti-inflammatory drugs
Warfarin
Intravenous heparin (rest pain/unstable angina)
Streptokinase/alteplase (t-PA)-thrombolytic therapy
Abciximab (Reopro)

*Impaired liver function*
Patients with abnormal clotting studies may require treatment to normalize these values, although this is not always appropriate (see section on drug therapy below). Liver function may well be depressed following cardiopulmonary by-pass and this can further impair the production of clotting factors. Significantly abnormal clotting studies which do not have a known aetiology require further investigation. Treatment of a known clotting defect can be categorized under the following headings:

1. Withdraw drug (e.g. aspirin) or reduce drug dosage (e.g. warfarin)
2. Administer fresh frozen plasma (FFP)
3. Administer vitamin K (caution – see below)
4. Administer platelets
5. Categorize and treat inherited coagulopathy (e.g. factor deficiency).

### Urea and electrolytes

Common abnormalities of urea and electrolytes are a low serum potassium due to chronic diuretic therapy and raised levels of serum urea and creatinine. In gross cardiac failure hyponatraemia can occur.

A chronically low serum potassium is not of concern unless the patient is on digoxin therapy, in which case digitalis toxicity is more likely. It is rarely necessary to acutely raise serum potassium levels prior to surgery and this may be risky. If time allows oral potassium supplements can be increased, otherwise it is safer to administer potassium during cardiopulmonary bypass (not in the pre-bypass period).

Elevated urea (>6.5 mmol/L) and creatinine (>120 mmol/L) levels should ring alarm bells to the cardiac anaesthetist because these levels are not raised until approximately 75% of renal function is lost. Renal failure is uncommon following cardiopulmonary bypass but once established carries a very high mortality. Monitoring urine output and renal function is essential in these high-risk patients. Measures that can be taken to prevent the onset of renal failure during the peri-operative period are summarized in Table 1.10.

### Liver function tests

Abnormalities of liver function usually relate to:

1. Heart failure (NB right heart failure with tricuspid incompetence)
2. Excessive alcohol intake.

Other causes of liver failure need further investigation.

Severe liver failure is very uncommon after cardiac surgery and pre-operative liver dysfunction is mainly of importance in relation to clotting abnormalities and

**Table 1.10 Measures to prevent onset of renal failure during peri-operative period**

Rehydrate prior to surgery
Limit period of starvation and fluid deprivation to a minimum pre-operatively (2 hours for fluid)
Re-hydrate prior to cardiopulmonary bypass
Add mannitol to pump prime
Consider low-dose dopamine (now controversial) or dopexamine
Maintain mean BP >60–70 mmHg post-bypass (higher if hypertensive)
Avoid use of NSAIDs and nephrotoxic drugs (especially antibiotics)

If above fails, consider:
  Frusemide infusion
  IV aminophylline
  IV urodilatin [atrial natiuretic peptide (ANF)]
  Haemofiltration

drug metabolism. Raised enzyme levels in an alcoholic patient also forewarn of general management problems in relation to the withdrawal of alcohol. This can be managed to some extent by the intravenous infusion of a low maintenance dose of absolute alcohol during the peri-operative period, given in aliquots in the hourly fluid maintenance.

### Blood glucose

A raised blood glucose may be found in a known diabetic or suggests previously undiscovered glucose intolerance. Many of these patients with a raised blood glucose will require intravenous insulin in the post-bypass period (12–24 hours) irrespective of whether they were receiving insulin, oral hypoglycaemics or no treatment pre-operatively. Normoglycaemia, with avoidance of hyperglycaemia, is optimal from the point of view of cerebral metabolism during CPB, but obviously hypoglycaemia should also be avoided.

## Specific cardiac investigations

### Electrocardiogram

The electrocardiogram (ECG) should be inspected for evidence of old or recent myocardial ischaemia, rhythm disturbances, ventricular hypertrophy or strain. Recent changes (e.g. worsening ischaemia or rhythm changes) are particularly relevant. The recording may be within normal limits but will still provide a useful baseline with which to compare postoperative records.

### Exercise electrocardiography

This procedure, often termed 'exercise testing', is particularly useful in the diagnosis and evaluation of ischaemic heart disease. There is an approximately linear increase in heart rate as myocardial oxygen consumption rises during exercise, and the duration of the exercise and the heart rate at the onset of ischaemic pain or ECG changes are reproducible indices of the severity of myocardial ischaemia. A positive exercise test (ST-segment depression equal to or greater than 1 mm, flat or downsloping, at 0.08 sec after the end of the S wave) aids diagnosis in patients with atypical chest pain and helps define the severity of coronary artery disease. With modern equipment a metabolic assessment of the patient's peak work load can also be made using maximum oxygen consumption ($VO_2$ max) measurements.

Most exercise testing is carried out on a treadmill where the gradient and speed can be increased progressively. Exercise testing should not be undertaken in patients with unstable angina, aortic stenosis, severe pulmonary hypertension or within 7 days of myocardial infarction. An experienced cardiologist should be present throughout the test. The Bruce protocol is often used but the modified Bruce protocol, which starts more slowly with gradual increases in gradient may be more appropriate in higher risk patients. There is a higher mortality among patients with comparable degree of coronary arterial disease if they have a positive exercise test and similar findings apply to those tested before discharge from hospital after myocardial infarction.

From the anaesthetic view point, a positive exercise test points to a higher risk patient, particularly if the test proved positive in the early stages of the protocol.

**Echocardiography**

Echocardiography now contributes to the diagnosis of most forms of cardiac disease although cardiac catheterization and angiography are still required to delineate coronary anatomy and some forms of congenital heart disease. There are two types of echocardiography, M-mode and two-dimensional or cross-sectional echocardiography. In M-mode echocardiography a single ultrasound beam is directed towards the heart. This technique is of particular value in diagnosing mitral and aortic valve disease and can be used to detect pericardial effusions, intracardiac tumours, left ventricular hypertrophy and left ventricular dysfunction. Multiple beams are used to create a sector-shaped cross-sectional image of the heart in two-dimensional echocardiography. Many frames are produced every minute and reproduced on a screen as a moving image. Views from several sites are used to build up a complete picture of the heart and therefore this technique is ideal for delineating differences in wall movement and complex anatomical relationships. Both types of echocardiography can be undertaken by the transthoracic or transoesophageal routes in most patients. Transoesophageal echocardiography (TOE) is becoming increasingly important in the intra-operative management of the cardiac surgical patient to assess repairs of congenital defects or valves, to image ventricular wall motion and to assess ventricular function. Doppler techniques (either continuous-wave or pulse-wave) are now widely applied during echocardiography to quantitate blood flow through intracardiac shunts and stenosed valves. Colour flow Doppler (via the TOE) is particularly useful in imaging regurgitant blood flow through valves at surgery and demonstrating residual septal defects.

At the pre-operative visit an anaesthetist will gain valuable information from any written summary of the echocardiographic findings. In the future it is likely that the majority of specialist cardiac anaesthetists will be able to use TOE intra-operatively and interpret the pre-operative findings independently.

## Cardiac catheterization and angiography

Accurate intracardiac pressure measurements can be obtained at cardiac catheterization along with values for oxygen saturation and oxygen content of the blood. If oxygen consumption is also measured, or taken from standard tables, a variety of other variables such as cardiac output, pulmonary to systemic blood flow ratios and pulmonary and systemic vascular resistance can be calculated. These are mainly of value in the evaluation of complex congenital heart disease, and possibly in the evaluation of end-stage valvular heart disease.

Angiography is used to delineate the anatomy and pathology of the coronary arteries (Fig. 1.1) and is sometimes used to demonstrate valvular and congenital defects when echocardiography has proved inconclusive. An angiogram taken with the radio-opaque dye injected rapidly into the left ventricle (ventriculogram) can be used to estimate ventricular function and ejection fraction. This latter value is calculated from the difference in ventricular size between systole and diastole and although it may only be calculated from one plane (coronary angiograms are usually taken in two planes) it is at least a reasonably objective measurement of ventricular function. The normal ejection fraction is approximately 70% and as this value drops with ventricular impairment the operative

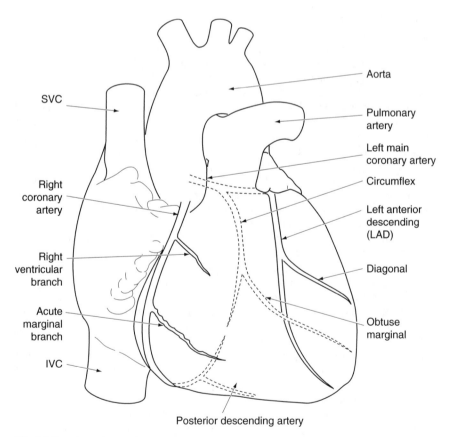

Fig. 1.1 Coronary artery anatomy

**Table 1.11 Cardiac catheter investigations – findings of particular relevance to anaesthesia**

*Angiography*
Congenital abnormalities
Valve lesions
  Stenosis
  Regurgitation
Ventricular function
  Presence of aneurysm
  Visualization of dyskinetic areas
  Ejection fraction measurement
Abnormalities of great vessels
  Acquired (e.g. dissecting aneurysm)
  Congenital (coarctation, vascular ring)

*Vascular and intracardiac pressure measurements*
Congenital abnormalities
Valve lesions
Ventricular function
  Atrial filling pressures
  Ventricular end-diastolic pressures

*Oxygen saturation/content measurements*
Diagnosis of congenital lesions – intra-cardiac shunts
Calculation of derived indices (see Table 1.12)

risk will increase for most procedures. Other determinants of left ventricular function which may be obtained at cardiac catheter include measurements of pre-load and after-load. Left atrial pressure (or pulmonary capillary wedge pressure – PCWP) and left ventricular end-diastolic pressure (LVEDP) represent pre-load. Systemic vascular resistance represents after-load.

The cardiac catheter findings should be available to the anaesthetist preoperatively and it is also instructive, where possible, to view angiograms that have been taken. The major points to note from the catheter report are summarized in Table 1.11 and derived indices with normal values are summarized in Table 1.12.

**Table 1.12 Derived indices**

| | |
|---|---|
| Cardiac output | CO |
| Cardiac index | CI = CO/Body surface area (BSA) |
| Stroke volume | SV = CO/Heart rate |
| Stroke volume index | SVI = SV/BSA |
| Pulmonary vascular resistance | PVR = (mean PAP − mean PCWP) × 80/CO |
| Systemic vascular resistance | SVR = (mean BP − mean RAP) × 80/CO |
| Left ventricular stroke work | LVSW = SV × (mean BP − mean PCWP) × 0.0136 |
| LV stroke work index | LVSWI = SVI × (mean BP − mean PCWP) × 0.0136 |

*Normal values*
CI   = 2.6–4.2 L/min/m$^2$
SVI  = 30–65 ml/beat/m$^2$
PVR  = 150–250 dynes.sec.cm$^{-5}$
SVR  = 700–1600 dynes.sec.cm$^{-5}$

PAP, pulmonary artery pressure; PCWP, pulmonary capillary wedge pressure; RAP, right atrial pressure

## Interventional cardiac catheterization techniques

In addition to diagnostic catheters many interventional procedures are now carried out under X-ray imaging in the catheter lab to treat cardiac lesions without resort to open operation. Angioplasty is used to ablate discrete coronary lesions with a balloon-dilatation catheter and stents may subsequently be inserted to maintain vessel patency. Balloon dilatation is also employed to treat pulmonary and aortic stenosis in children and certain types of aortic and mitral valve stenosis in adults. In the paediatric field closure of the patent ductus arteriosus is now a routine procedure in the catheter laboratory and it is becoming more common to close simple intra-atrial and ventricular defects with a device inserted via a catheter. A full discussion of interventional cardiology and the increasingly complex field of electrophysiology is beyond the scope of this book. The anaesthetist is most likely to become involved in these procedures, however, when complications occur necessitating emergency surgery. The anaesthetic management of failed angioplasty is discussed in subsequent chapters.

## Nuclear cardiological investigations

Myocardial perfusion imaging with radiotracers is now increasingly used in the patient with ischaemic heart disease particularly to assess myocardial viability in ischaemic left ventricular dysfunction. A radiotracer such as thallium-201 (or more recently SESTAMIBI labelled with technetium-99m) is injected intravenously and distributes in proportion to regional cardiac output. Hypoperfused areas in the heart will appear as image defects, when visualized with the gamma camera, in comparison with normally perfused areas.

This type of myocardial perfusion scanning is often carried out during exercise and then some time later at rest. Thus if the 'stress' perfusion scan demonstrates an area of hypoperfused myocardium which then recovers during rest it can be assumed that there is viable myocardium supplied by a diseased coronary artery. This is particularly useful information in a patient with poor ventricular function because it could be expected that revascularization of the appropriate coronary vessels in this situation may improve myocardial contractility. The 'stress' on the myocardium can also be produced pharmacologically with dypyridamole, adenosine or dobutamine. Dypiridamole and adenosine increase coronary blood flow and seem to produce a 'coronary steal' effect in favour of the normal coronary arteries, thereby creating a perfusion defect in the myocardium supplied by diseased arteries. Dobutamine, particularly at high doses, creates a significant increase in blood pressure and heart rate and myocardial perfusion scanning in this context has been shown to have a high sensitivity and specificity for detecting ischaemic heart disease.

The main question in an anaesthetist's mind when confronted with the results of a myocardial perfusion scan, particularly in a patient with a low ejection fraction, should be, 'Does this patient have recoverable and viable myocardium?'

## Computed tomography (CT) and magnetic resonance imaging (MRI)

CT and MRI are particularly useful in imaging the thoracic aorta and detecting aortic dissection. Either technique may be useful in assessing the risks involved in opening the chest surgically for re-operations, specifically imaging the position of the heart and great vessels in relation to the sternum. MRI has also been used to assess graft patency after coronary artery surgery.

# Drug therapy

The management of current drug therapy in the patient presenting for cardiac surgery can be a daunting problem for the inexperienced. In practice a few sensible guidelines can be employed to overcome many of the potential therapeutic difficulties, although as further knowledge accumulates these will, of necessity, change from time to time. The relevance of cardiac drug therapy to the peri-operative period is discussed below. The management of general drug therapy is beyond the scope of this chapter.

## Anticoagulants

### Aspirin

Many patients with coronary artery disease will be taking aspirin prior to surgery because it has been shown that its anti-platelet effect reduces mortality and infarction rates in unstable angina and significantly decreases vascular mortality in acute myocardial infarction. Aspirin permanently inactivates the enzyme cyclo-oxygenase by acetylation and thereby prevents the formation of platelet-activating thromboxane $A_2$. The action of aspirin is normally as long as the lifetime of the affected platelets in the circulation.

In a stable patient with coronary artery disease it is usual to stop oral aspirin therapy at least 1 week prior to surgery in order to allow new platelets with normal function to reappear in the circulation. Platelet function is depressed following cardiopulmonary bypass in any event and the additional effect of aspirin leads to increased bleeding with a higher incidence of re-opening the chest ('re-sternotomy') to manage postoperative bleeding surgically. If the patient has unstable angina and/or a critical coronary lesion such as left main stem stenosis it is probably safer, however, to continue aspirin therapy up until the time of surgery. In this situation the risk of excessive postoperative bleeding can be minimized by careful haemostasis and the infusion of platelets (usually a 5–6 unit donor pack). Aprotinin therapy also reduces the incidence of postoperative bleeding in patients on aspirin but its use remains somewhat controversial in those presenting for coronary artery surgery. Many surgeons believe this therapy may adversely effect graft patency. This view is not confirmed, however, in the majority of reported studies.

Aspirin improves graft patency rates following coronary artery surgery and is commonly prescribed as long-term treatment postoperatively.

### Non-steroidal anti-inflammatory drugs (NSAIDs)

Non-steroidal anti-inflammatory drugs such as ibuprofen and diclofenac sodium act in a similar fashion to aspirin and inhibit the prostaglandin-forming cyclo-oxygenase.

They are widely used as anti-inflammatory agents and many patients referred for cardiac surgery will be taking these drugs for reasons quite unrelated to their cardiac status. These drugs also have an adverse effect on platelet function and, if symptoms allow, they should be stopped 1 week to 10 days before cardiac surgery. It is relatively common, however, for patients to remain on NSAIDs, almost by default, when aspirin therapy has been stopped. If this is the case and the patient has already been admitted for surgery it is common practice to proceed to surgery knowing there may be an increased risk of postoperative bleeding (although this appears to be less well documented than with aspirin). It is our practice to order platelets for transfusion, in advance, if either there is visual evidence of excess bleeding at sternotomy or if the procedure is relatively complex (such as a re-operation or valve replacement combined with coronary grafting). A lower threshold for platelet therapy also appears reasonable in the elderly when the concerns regarding transfusion-related problems are out-weighed clinically by the considerable morbidity, if not mortality, associated with re-opening for postoperative bleeding in this age group.

NSAIDs cause gastrointestinal side effects similar to aspirin and also impairment of renal function. This latter problem may either be of a chronic nature due to an interstitial nephritis or an acute event due to suppression of renal vasodilator prostaglandin synthesis. If there is evidence of mild to moderate renal impairment NSAIDs should be stopped pre-operatively and the precautions detailed in Table 1.10 taken during the peri-operative period. If marked renal impairment is present pre-operatively the opinion of a renal physician should be sought prior to surgery. The problem of acute renal failure due to NSAIDs is not uncommon when these drugs are given to supplement analgesia in the postoperative period. In essence they should not be given to patients postoperatively if there is any evidence of impaired renal function pre-operatively, or if there is excess bleeding. These drugs should also be used cautiously in the elderly. If renal function is affected urine output is usually re-established with fluid loading (where appropriate) and the administration of an intravenous diuretic, with or without the addition of low-dose dopamine. No further NSAIDs should be given (see also Chapter 5 for a discussion on the treatment of postoperative renal impairment).

### Warfarin

Warfarin, a synthetic coumarin derivative, is the most widely used oral anticoagulant. Warfarin acts by preventing the formation of active coagulation factors II, VII, IX and X in the liver by inhibiting the vitamin-K-mediated gamma carboxylation of the precursor proteins. Cardiac surgery patients may be taking warfarin for a variety of reasons including the presence of a prosthetic valve, chronic atrial fibrillation, pulmonary emboli and the adjunctive management of coronary occlusion. The activity of warfarin is monitored by the prothrombin time (PT) in individuals, but the recommended international normalized ratio (INR) seems to vary from condition to condition and even between different institutions. The target INR is in the region of 3.0 to 3.5 for a mitral valve prosthesis and possibly slightly lower for an aortic prosthesis.

It is routine practice to withdraw warfarin in treated individuals prior to cardiac surgery in such a manner as to reduce the INR to between 2 and 2.5 on the day of surgery. If there is particular concern regarding thromboembolism associated with a prosthetic valve or a severe coronary lesion, for example, then intravenous heparin therapy can be commenced to cover the operative period.

If the INR is initially high, despite withdrawal of warfarin, surgery may have to be delayed. Alternatively the effect of warfarin can be reversed with the administration of vitamin $K_1$ (phytonadione) or fresh frozen plasma (FFP) at an effective volume of 10 to 20 ml/kg.

Vitamin $K_1$ reverses the effect of warfarin via the synthesis of fully carboxylated coagulation proteins in the liver and, regardless of the route of administration, significant improvement in the coagulation profile may not occur for several hours and may take 24 hours or longer. The effect of vitamin K is irreversible, however, and should be avoided if another prosthetic valve is to be inserted. The administration of FFP is a preferable treatment. This provides a source of the vitamin-K-dependent coagulation factors and has an immediate effect. Further amounts of FFP may be required after cardiopulmonary bypass because in normal circumstances these transfused factors, particularly factor VII, are cleared from the circulation more quickly than is the residual oral anticoagulant. In addition, during cardiopulmonary bypass, levels of clotting factors decline further and platelet activity is inhibited.

## Heparin

Heparin acts indirectly at multiple sites in the clotting cascade to potentiate the inhibitory action of anti-thrombin III. It also prevents the formation of a fibrin clot by inhibiting the thrombin-activated formation of fibrin-stabilizing factor. Intravenous heparin improves coronary patency after acute myocardial infarction and is an effective treatment of unstable angina, when it is usually given together with an infusion of glyceryl trinitrate (GTN). Patients with unstable angina may be receiving intravenous heparin, by continuous infusion, pre-operatively. This infusion should be kept running up until the loading dose of heparin is given prior to cardiopulmonary bypass. Heparin resistance may occur in these patients and this is probably due to low anti-thrombin III levels. Increased doses of heparin usually raise the activated clotting time above the required 480 sec but it has been found empirically that the administration of FFP decreases heparin requirements to the normal range, presumably because it is a source of anti-thrombin III.

## Thrombolytic agents

Thrombolytic agents such as streptokinase and alteplase (tissue-type plasminogen activator or t-PA) increase the amount of plasmin available locally to break down fresh clot. These agents are therefore widely used systemically to lyse clots which may be forming, or have formed, within the coronary arteries during the course of myocardial infarction or unstable angina.

Patients occasionally present for surgery after recent thrombolytic therapy, usually following a failed angioplasty or coronary stent procedure. Most thrombolytic drugs have a short half-life varying from 5–15 min, apart from anistreplase (APSAC) but, nevertheless, heparinization increases the ever-present risk of pathological bleeding in this group of patients. Bleeding following cardiopulmonary bypass can usually be managed with infusion of the appropriate clotting factors contained in FFP and cryoprecipitate. Protease inhibitors such as epsilon-aminocaproic acid (EACA) and aprotinin, which inhibit fibrinolysis, may also have a role to play in the postoperative haemostatic process although, in general, they should be used with caution. Aprotinin inhibits both kallikrein and plasmin, and by inhibiting plasmin it protects platelets, blocks fibrinolysis and decreases production of fibrin degradation products (FDPs) during cardiopulmonary bypass.

### Newer anti-platelet agents

Platelet aggregation is an important factor in the development of a thrombus after arterial injury. Prevention of platelet aggregation is, therefore, an important therapeutic manoeuvre in a number of clinical situations such as acute myocardial infarction, unstable angina and the coronary interventions of angioplasty and stenting. Newer drugs are being developed to prevent platelet aggregation and abciximab (Reopro, Lilly) has recently been licensed for use in the UK.

Abciximab is a monoclonal antibody to the glycoprotein IIb/IIIa receptor which is expressed on the surface of activated platelets. Expression of this receptor is the final common pathway in platelet aggregation and blocking the receptor with abciximab prevents platelet aggregation more effectively than conventional agents such as aspirin. Abciximab is used intravenously during high-risk angioplasty and coronary stent insertion. Anaesthetists will, therefore, be required to deal with the adverse effects of abciximab in patients proceeding to surgery after failed procedures. Excessive bleeding is obviously of most concern, although in recent trials (EPIC, 1994 and EPILOG, 1997) those patients requiring urgent bypass surgery following angioplasty did not have significantly higher bleeding or transfusion requirements whether on placebo or abciximab. Abciximab, however, continues to occupy the IIb/IIIa binding sites for approximately 36–48 hours after an infusion is stopped and platelet aggregation is inhibited for at least 72 hours. Abciximab can also cause thrombocytopenia. In the light of these facts it is perhaps not surprising that many surgeons report (anecdotally) that excess bleeding does occur with abciximab. In any event clinicians should be prepared for increased transfusion requirements if surgery is planned and, most importantly, ensure there is a plentiful supply of fresh donor platelets available.

Ticlopidine is another anti-platelet agent which is currently used in North America and many European countries and may be introduced into the UK in the near future. This drug is given orally to prevent platelet aggregation. It is structurally unrelated to other currently available platelet aggregation inhibitors and is thought to work via the inhibition of adenosine diphosphate (ADP)-induced platelet aggregation. There are many adverse effects associated with the use of ticlopidine. Excess intra-operative bleeding is an obvious risk in patients taking ticlopidine and, where possible, patients should stop taking the drug 10–14 days prior to surgery. If this cannot be achieved platelet transfusion will be required. In addition to its effect on platelet aggregation ticlopidine may cause thrombocytopenia and neutropenia. Neutropenia occurs in up to 2% of patients on long-term therapy. The white cell count usually returns to normal within 1–3 weeks of discontinuing ticlopidine but rare fatalities have been reported. In patients undergoing cardiac surgery, with its related immunosuppression, neutropenia poses a major risk as far as infection is concerned. Surgery should, therefore, be postponed, if at all possible, until the white cell count has returned to the normal range.

## Cardiovascular drugs

The majority of drugs used to improve a patient's cardiovascular status should be continued up to (and including) the morning of surgery. There are a few exceptions to this general rule, for example beta-adrenergic blocking drugs are normally withheld in the presence of a severe bradycardia, and these are detailed below.

### Beta-adrenergic blocking agents

Beta-adrenergic blocking agents (beta-blockers) are used to treat hypertension and angina and have been shown to reduce mortality following myocardial infarction. In cardiac patients with ischaemic heart disease it is preferable to continue beta-blockade up to the time of operation to prevent peri-operative ischaemia and hypertension. Some clinicians restart beta-blockade in the postoperative period, in those patients with good ventricular function, to control hypertension and also as prophylaxis against atrial dysrhythmias.

The main disadvantage to beta-blockade in the peri-operative period is the possibility of exaggerated cardiac effects giving rise to bradycardia, heart block and even myocardial failure. If marked bradycardia (less than 40 beats per minute) is present pre-operatively the drugs may be tailed off, bearing in mind the different half-lives of the various drugs. Bradycardia can be treated intra-operatively with atropine, intravenous dobutamine or epicardial pacing. Iso-prenaline should be used with extreme caution in patients with ischaemic heart disease because it lowers the diastolic blood pressure ($beta_2$ effect – relaxation of vascular smooth muscle) and may compromise coronary perfusion.

### Nitrates

Nitrates provide a source of nitric oxide (NO) to vascular cells. They are effective coronary vasodilators and also produce peripheral venous dilatation and a decrease in myocardial oxygen demand. Nitrates are, in general, well tolerated. They are administered via a variety of routes in the form of glyceryl trinitrate (nitroglycerine), isosorbide dinitrate or isosorbide mononitrate and should be continued in normal dosage up to the time of surgery. This should include any oral dose due on the morning of surgery and also the continuation of an intravenous infusion at least until full monitoring has been established prior to the induction of anaesthesia.

### Calcium antagonists

The calcium antagonists are a chemically heterogeneous group of drugs used in the treatment of angina and hypertension, mainly because of their coronary and peripheral vasodilator effects. These drugs do have some negative inotropic effect which is most marked with verapamil. Verapamil is mainly used as an anti-dysrhythmic drug, however, because of its inhibitory action on the atrio-venticular (AV) node, a property which nifedipine lacks. Calcium antagonists should be used with care in combination with beta-blockers because there may be an additive negative inotropic effect leading to myocardial failure. In practice the safer drugs such as nifedipine are often used in combination with beta-blockers and nitrates.

Calcium antagonists should be continued up until the time of operation unless there are signs of myocardial failure or significant prolongation of the PR interval on the ECG. Abrupt withdrawal of these drugs can, however, cause rebound angina in patients with ischaemic heart disease and this should be avoided where possible.

Intra-operatively calcium antagonists appear 'benign' and potential drug interactions such as the potentiation of hypotension with the administration of cimetidine and the prolongation of action of neuromuscular blockers are rarely of practical importance.

## Potassium channel opening drugs

Nicorandil is the first potassium channel opener combined with a nitrate available in the UK for the treatment of angina. Its anti-anginal effects are mediated by its ability to relax vascular smooth muscle and it dilates both normal and stenotic segments of coronary arteries. It also dilates systemic veins and arteries reducing pre-load and after-load but there are no direct effects on myocardial contractility or heart rate, apart from a slight reflex tachycardia at high doses.

Nicorandil appears to have few side effects, apart from headache, and it can be used safely with other anti-anginals, digoxin and frusemide. On basis of the principles previously discussed oral potassium channel openers should be continued up to the time of surgery. There is little information available regarding the use of potassium channel openers in the intra-operative period but they have a potential cardioprotective effect and may reduce post-ischaemia reperfusion injury. An intravenous preparation, which could also be added to cardioplegic solution, is not yet available in the UK.

## Angiotensin converting enzyme inhibitors

Angiotensin converting enzyme (ACE) inhibitors, such as captopril and enalapril, are widely used in the treatment of hypertension and congestive heart failure. They are particularly effective in reducing blood pressure in combination with low-dose thiazide diuretics, in which case they offset potential hypokalaemia. ACE inhibitors may, however, cause hyperkalaemia if used in conjunction with potassium sparing diuretics or if co-administered with potassium supplements. They have an additive anti-hypertensive effect if combined with calcium antagonists, but less so with beta-blockers. In hypertensives with renal failure ACE inhibitors may improve renal function but, on the other hand, undue hypotension may have a deleterious effect on renal function.

ACE inhibitor therapy is usually continued up until the time of surgery to prevent the occurrence of rebound hypertension. The last dose of longer acting drugs such as enalapril (plasma half-life 11 hours) could, however, be safely omitted. There is some concern, however, and a certain amount of evidence, that ACE inhibitors may contribute to an unacceptable level of hypotension during and after cardiopulmonary bypass in individual patients. If hypotension does occur in patients taking ACE inhibitors it is sometimes necessary to give quite large doses of vasoconstrictors (e.g. metaraminol, phenylephrine or noradrenaline), particularly during bypass, in order to restore the systemic vascular resistance. In the post-bypass period appropriate fluid loading will also be required. In extreme cases of hypotension it may be necessary to administer angiotensin intravenously.

## Anti-dysrhythmic drugs, diuretics and lipid lowering agents

The above drugs are not generally withdrawn prior to surgery and may need to be continued postoperatively.

Binding of digoxin may be affected by cardiopulmonary bypass and in the past it was traditional to withdraw the drug a few days before surgery. If digoxin levels are within the therapeutic range this step is no longer deemed necessary, particularly as serum potassium levels can easily and regularly be measured on modern analysers within the theatre suite. If digoxin levels are within the toxic range prior to emergency cardiac surgery it is possible to treat this effectively with digoxin binding fraction (Digibind). This treatment makes subsequent digoxin level measurements uninterpretable, however.

## Hypoglycaemic drugs

Diabetic patients presenting for cardiac surgery can be managed on general principles applicable to other forms of major surgery carried out under general anaesthesia. Requirements for insulin and oral hypoglycaemics will be decreased in the immediate pre-operative period, particularly if the patient is spending more time resting than usual, and dosages should be curtailed appropriately. The period of starvation prior to routine surgery should be kept to a minimum in uncomplicated cases. We allow a traditional English 'early morning cup of tea' (or other beverage of choice) in all adult patients approximately 2 hours prior to surgery and a light breakfast if surgery is not scheduled for 3–5 hours.

Many known diabetics will require insulin during the peri-operative period even if controlled by oral hypoglycaemics or diet pre-operatively. In addition, it is not uncommon for patients with even moderate glucose intolerance to require insulin in the first 12 hours or so following surgery, as a result of the increased stress of operation and cardiopulmonary bypass. In either case a simple 'sliding-scale' infusion of soluble insulin combined with dextrose-containing intravenous fluid replacement will control blood glucose levels satisfactorily in the majority of cases. Insulin requirements tend to decrease significantly after the initial 12–24-hour period and then patients can usually be weaned back to their pre-operative treatment regime.

## Premedication

Traditionally heavy premedication was prescribed prior to surgery for ischaemic heart disease in order to prevent the onset of angina before and during induction of anaesthesia. Medical control of ischaemia has improved substantially over the last few years, however, and if drug therapy is continued up to the time of surgery there is no longer a requirement for heavy sedation. There is also some concern that a number of patients will become relatively hypoxic when over-sedated pre-operatively unless supplemental oxygen is administered. Heavy premedication with long-acting drugs may also may be a factor in delaying planned early extubation in 'fast-track' patients.

We currently prescribe the relatively short-acting benzodiazepine temazepam prior to surgery. A dose of 10–20 mg is given orally 2 hours before surgery, but if the starting time of operation is unclear (for organizational or other reasons) we give oral temazepam at 7.00 am and repeat this at 4–6 hourly intervals as appropriate.

Premedication obviously has to be tailored to individual patients' needs and in the elderly or frail (often scheduled for valvular heart surgery) it may be necessary to decrease dosage or omit sedative drugs altogether.

Other premedicant drugs used before cardiac surgery include morphine or papaveretum given, combined with hyoscine, intramuscularly 1–2 hours before induction. Diazepam and lorazepam are also used as oral premedication but, as outlined above, we tend to avoid the longer-acting benzodiazepines.

### Antibiotic prophylaxis

Prophylactic antibiotics are given to cover all forms of cardiac surgery. The first dose of antibiotic is usually given intravenously in the anaesthetic room and ideally this should be given before catheterization of the bladder in patients with valvular heart disease.

Dosage regimes and the choice of antibiotic vary from unit to unit. Theoretically, effective surgical antibiotic prophylaxis only requires adequate tissue levels of drug at the time of operation but in practice many surgeons continue antibiotics for up to 36 or even 48 hours postoperatively. Following cardiac surgery this may be justifiable, however, because of the presence of central venous lines, chest drains and so on. In routine practice antibiotics are discontinued after 48 hours at the latest but if the postoperative course is complicated further therapy will require careful review based on the clinical condition of the patient and the results of relevant bacteriological investigations.

The choice of antibiotic for prophylaxis is problematical. We use a first generation cephalosporin such as cephazolin for routine coronary surgery. This agent is simple to administer, is not nephrotoxic and provides better anti-staphylococcal cover than third generation agents. For cover during valve surgery we use flucloxacillin and gentamicin, unless these drugs are contraindicated. After homograft aortic valve replacement teicoplanin and fucidin are given for a period of 5 days. This latter regime is intended to prevent aortic root infection and guard against the remote possibility that the homograft, despite prior treatment, is harbouring viable organisms.

## References

Campeau IL. (1975) Grading of angina pectoris. *Circulation;* **54:** 522.

EPIC Investigators (1994) Use of a monoclonal antibody directed against the platelet glycoprotein IIb/IIIa receptor in high risk coronary angioplasty. *N Engl J Med;* **330:** 956–961.

EPILOG Investigators (1997) Platelet IIb/IIIa receptor blockade and low-dose heparin during percutaneous coronary revascularization. *N Engl J Med;* **336:** 1689–1696.

Parsonnet V., Dean D. and Bernstein A.D. (1989) A method of uniform stratification of risk for evaluating the results of surgery in acquired adult heart disease. *Circulation;* **79** (suppl 1): 1.3–1.12.

Stedmon J., Yentis S.S., Levinson A. and Morgan C. (1995) Comparison of two different scoring systems for predicting outcome after cardiac surgery. *Br J Anaesth;* **74:** 488P.

# Further reading

Mangano D.T. (1990) *Preoperative Cardiac Assessment. A Society of Cardiovascular Anesthesiologists Monograph.* J.B. Lippincott, Philadelphia.

Miller G.A.H. (1990) *Handbook of Cardiac Catheterisation.* Blackwell Scientific Publications, Oxford.

Millner R. and Treasure T. (1995) *Explaining Cardiac Surgery. Patient Assessment and Care.* BMJ, London.

Vlay S.C. (1992) *Medical Care of the Cardiac Surgical Patient.* Blackwell Scientific Publications, Boston.

Chapter 2

# Anaesthesia for cardiac surgery

## Introduction

There are now a large number of accepted anaesthetic techniques applicable to cardiac surgery. New drugs continue to be developed and introduced into clinical practice so that there is bound to be a diversity of opinion as to the optimal anaesthetic for a particular cardiac procedure. Fortunately there is substantial evidence that it is not the initial choice of a particular anaesthetic technique or group of drugs which is crucial to outcome but rather the manner in which these techniques and drugs are applied in different clinical circumstances. Reves *et al.* (1995) in a recent editorial, stated:

> '. . . the point is that drugs with very different sites and mechanisms of action can be given to achieve the same hemodynamic and other efficacy end-points during cardiac anesthesia.'

They went on to conclude that there is no such entity as a 'cardiac anaesthetic' and that what is required to anaesthetize patients with ischaemic heart disease is knowledge of the pathophysiology of the disease and of the clinical pharmacology of any number of anaesthetic vasoactive drugs at the practioner's disposal. The outcome of surgery for ischaemic heart disease may be influenced by the manner in which anaesthesia is conducted, but of paramount importance is that the surgeon achieves adequate revascularization without significantly impairing myocardial function.

It is impossible to describe in detail the pharmacology and cardiovascular effects of all the commonly used anaesthetic drugs in a short chapter of this nature. A description of the techniques and drug therapy we currently use in different circumstances is therefore set out below and where appropriate the possible advantages and disadvantages of different anaesthetic approaches are discussed. The relevant cardiovascular effects of the major induction agents, inhalational agents and muscle relaxants are provided in tabular form (Tables 2.5–2.7).

The first part of this chapter covers intra-operative monitoring, induction and maintenance of anaesthesia and haemodynamic management for adult cardiac surgery in general terms. Management of problems relating to specific types of cardiac surgery and clinical circumstances are described in more detail in Chapter 3.

**Table 2.1 Standard monitoring for cardiopulmonary bypass**

Pulse oximetry
Inspired/expired gas analysis: $CO_2/O_2$/inhalational agent
Tidal volume/inflation pressure (minimum requirement)

Nasopharyngeal temperature
Peripheral temperature
Myocardial temperature

Urine output

Electrocardiogram (4 leads, plus V5)

Arterial pressure
Central venous pressure
Pulmonary artery pressure (intermittent pulmonary capillary wedge pressure)

Cardiac output – thermodilution

Other techniques
  Transoesophageal echocardiography
  Cerebral function monitoring

# Monitoring

Monitoring techniques for cardiopulmonary bypass now differ little from unit to unit. These are summarized in Table 2.1. Before anaesthesia a four lead electrocardiogram (ECG) plus V5 chest lead is attached to the patient and monitored. Additional non-invasive monitoring should include oxygen saturation measurement, end-tidal oxygen, carbon dioxide and inhalational agent analysis and, prior to arterial cannulation, a cuff blood pressure measurement. Consideration can then be given to the more invasive and/or complex modes of monitoring discussed below.

## Arterial cannulation

An arterial cannula (20 gauge) is usually inserted percutaneously under local anaesthesia in the radial artery prior to the induction of anaesthesia. The arterial wave form is then displayed. This is mandatory in high-risk cases such as severe aortic stenosis and left main stem coronary artery stenosis.

A test of ulnar artery collateral blood flow, such as a modified Allen's test, should be carried out prior to cannulation of the radial artery if there is doubt about blood supply to the hand, for example because of previous injury, or if an aberrant artery is palpable. This type of test is no longer carried out on a routine basis in many units. The very low incidence of major complications following radial artery cannulation probably reflects improved expertise in placement and, more importantly, the design and manufacture of modern cannulae, disposable transducers and flushing systems. It is prudent not to be too complacent, however, and the skin of the lower arm and hand should be inspected for discoloration on a regular basis in the postoperative period.

It is common practice to cannulate the left radial artery prior to coronary artery surgery and this does have the advantage that it is the non-dominant hand in the majority of patients. The arterial trace from a left radial artery line is occasionally obliterated as the subclavian artery is stretched by the overzealous use of a sternal retractor during dissection of the left internal mammary artery. For this reason some anaesthetists use the right radial artery for their primary site of cannulation in patients scheduled for coronary surgery, as in routine practice the right internal mammary artery is less commonly used as a vascular conduit. The right radial artery is also preferred if aortic surgery is planned and for the purposes of timing intra-aortic balloon pump (IABP) counter pulsation by certain surgeons. In addition, if the radial artery is to be used as a vascular conduit for coronary artery bypass surgery it is usually taken from the non-dominant arm. As this is commonly the left side it has the added advantage that the internal mammary artery can be dissected out simultaneously by a second surgeon standing at the right-hand side of the operating table.

In adolescents and small women a 22 gauge cannula is sometimes easier to site than a 20 gauge cannula and still provides a satisfactory waveform. If it is difficult to thread an arterial cannula up the radial artery, after a satisfactory flash-back of blood has been realized via a syringe, a fine guide wire can be an invaluable aid.

If radial artery cannulation proves impossible percutaneously it is inadvisable to try to cannulate the ulnar artery. This is likely to compromise blood supply to the hand. There are a number of other possible sites for arterial cannulation including axillary, dorsalis pedis, brachial and femoral arteries. The dorsalis pedis pulse can be satisfactorily cannulated in a number of patients. This artery may not be easily palpable in a patient with aortic stenosis or a poor cardiac output, however, and will give a poor trace when the patient is peripherally cold. The brachial and femoral arteries can be cannulated percutaneously but there is not an extensive collateral circulation at these sites, hence there is an increased risk of limb ischaemia. A femoral artery site may also be required for IABP insertion or femoral cannulation to establish cardiopulmonary bypass. As a last resort a surgical 'cut-down' can be carried out and a cannula inserted into the radial artery under direct vision. This is rarely necessary.

### Central venous access

Peripheral venous access will obviously be gained prior to induction of anaesthesia in all patients and a large bore cannula can be used for volume replacement during surgery, if required. This peripheral infusion site will not be available for inspection during surgery and there is the small possibility that large volumes of fluid might be transfused into the tissues in error, particularly if a pressure infusion device is used. For this reason we prefer to rely on central venous infusion sites for transfusion (and administration of vasoactive drugs) during surgery.

Central venous access for central venous pressure (CVP) measurement and transfusion is more easily achieved after induction of anaesthesia in the routine case but can be established under local anaesthetic in the high risk patient. The preferred route for central venous cannulation is the right internal jugular vein. This is easier to cannulate than the left internal jugular vein and pressure recordings are not affected if the innominate vein is stretched when the chest is opened. The subclavian vein is an alternative site but this is generally considered more hazardous in the context of inadvertent arterial puncture, pneumothorax and heparinization for cardiopulmonary bypass.

Since the original description of internal jugular cannulation by English *et al.* in 1969 many different techniques have been published. The 'higher' approaches to the internal jugular are preferable because pneumothorax or damage to vascular structures within the chest is less likely. In general it is safer to use a Seldinger technique, locating the vein with a relatively fine needle or cannula initially, and then introducing a larger cannula with the aid of a guide wire. Multi-lumen catheters are ideal for cardiac surgery when placed in this way and a quadruple or triple-lumen cannula can be used in the right internal jugular vein in combination with a pulmonary artery catheter (PAC) sheath for more complex cases.

The 'educated hand' can usually palpate the internal jugular vein, particularly in the anaesthetized and paralysed patient in a head-down position. This is our preferred method of locating the vein but others use anatomical landmarks such as the position of the two heads of the sternomastoid muscle or the carotid artery to estimate its position. Small purpose-made ultrasound probes are available to detect the position of the internal jugular vein and this can be invaluable if other methods prove unhelpful. Practical hints to facilitate internal jugular cannulation are listed in Table 2.2.

Major complications of internal jugular cannulation including pneumothorax and arterial puncture are rare, but can have catastrophic consequences. Carotid artery puncture is not usually a serious matter if the artery is 'hit' in the neck, although one is always concerned that coronary patients may have an unknown degree of atheromatous carotid disease. Firm pressure on the neck after withdrawal of the needle will prevent anything other than moderate haematoma formation, even with later heparinization, in the majority of cases. It is possible to lacerate the carotid and/or subclavian arteries if blind, rash, attempts are made to cannulate the internal vein low in the neck. Rarely, this may be a cause of intra- or postoperative bleeding which is difficult to see and therefore appreciate and, because of poor access, even more difficult to repair surgically.

**Table 2.2 Internal jugular cannulation – practicalities**

Try to palpate the internal jugular vein (IJV) once the patient is anaesthetized and paralysed

Place the patient head down. Approx 15° of head-down tilt is usually optimal. Excessive head-down tilt causes unnecessary venous engorgement which may compromise cerebral blood flow

Do *not* hyperextend the patient's neck. This will only narrow the IJV

Place the head in a neutral position but with the head turned away from the side of cannulation. Avoid excessive rotation, however

The IJV is usually (but not always) lateral to the carotid artery

Avoid digital pressure on the carotid artery when attempting to cannulate the IJV. This will only narrow the IJV

If location of the IJV proves difficult use a fine 'seeker' needle before attempting with a larger bore needle or cannula

## Pulmonary artery catheterization

The routine use of pulmonary artery catheters (PACs) remains a controversial area in relation to cardiac surgery. PA catheterization allows measurement of pulmonary artery pressure, pulmonary capillary wedge pressure (PCWP – which in most circumstances relates to left atrial pressure) and, in the specialized forms of the catheter, permits measurement of thermodilution cardiac output and continuous mixed venous oxygen saturation. A variety of haemodynamic indices can then be calculated from these data and other less complex measurements of systolic/diastolic blood pressure and central venous pressure (see Chapter 1, Table 1.12 for derived indices). In patients with ventricular failure the measurement of both right and left heart filling pressures can be invaluable, but at operation left-sided pressures can be measured using a left atrial line or, more simply, with a fine needle temporarily inserted into the left atrium and connected to a pressure transducer. Much information can also be gained by observing the contraction and filling state of the right and left heart and the pulmonary artery without recourse to invasive PA monitoring. Additional evidence of cardiac performance can be documented by intra-operative transoesophageal echocardiography (TOE) as discussed below.

Several centres have reported excellent surgical results without the universal utilization of PACs or with no use of them at all in patients undergoing routine coronary artery surgery (Liban and Davies, 1986). Inserting PACs in all patients undergoing cardiac surgery is a practice advocated by certain North American centres, whereas in the UK very few centres have, in the past, placed PACs for routine cases. This divergence of opinion has become much less over recent years as American centres have become more aware of the complications (see Table 2.3) and costs of routine PAC placement, and UK anaesthetists have become more aware of their value in managing the high-risk case.

A study by Tuman *et al.* (1989a) gives some credence to this change in attitude. These authors prospectively investigated the occurrence of complications and outcome of cardiac surgery in 1094 consecutive patients monitored, irrespective of cardiac risk, with either elective PACs (537 patients) or central venous pressure monitoring (557 patients). No significant difference in any of the outcome variables was noted between any groups of patients with similar risk factors. A group of 39 patients monitored initially with central venous pressure only were thought to require PAC monitoring during the study because of the occurrence of major haemodynamic events. Late utilization of PAC monitoring in this group did not affect outcome variables when compared with a similar group of patients monitored with PACs from the outset.

**Table 2.3 Complications of pulmonary artery catheters**

Infection
Thrombosis or embolism
Rhythm disturbances
Pulmonary haemorrhage
Pulmonary artery disruption
Knotting of catheter
Pneumothorax/vascular damage during insertion

On the basis of these findings it seems reasonable to confine pulmonary artery catheterization to patients in a high-risk category, particularly those with poor left ventricular function. An alternative approach is to place an introducer sheath for the PAC into the internal jugular vein at induction of anaesthesia. A PAC can then be easily introduced, when required, during the procedure or at a later stage in the intensive care unit when serial measurements of haemodynamic indices can be invaluable in the management of patients with a marginal cardiac output.

## Transoesophageal echocardiography

The use of intra-operative transoesophageal echocardiography (TOE) is likely to become commonplace in the next few years, as discussed in Chapter 1. We are now used to cardiologists providing intra-operative TOE services to aid surgery such as valve repair and the correction of congenital defects and also to facilitate weaning from cardiopulmonary bypass when difficulties arise. In North America and certain European centres anaesthetists themselves are extensively involved in the provision of intra-operative diagnosis with TOE. Despite the high cost of the equipment and the need for adequate training and cardiological/technical support it is likely that cardiac anaesthetists in the UK will increasingly take on this role.

**Table 2.4 Intra-operative transoesophageal echocardiography (TOE)**

*Advantages*
Non-invasive, low-risk procedure
Good image quality
Does not interfere with surgery
Continuous monitor of myocardial function

*Indications*
Valve repair
Valve replacement (especially of the homografts/stentless valves )
Known myocardial/valvular dysfunction
Risk of myocardial ischaemia
Congenital heart disease
Difficulty in weaning from CPB

*Uses*
Assessment of global/regional myocardial function
Monitoring myocardial ischaemia (regional wall motion abnormalities)
Assessment of ventricular filling
Evaluating surgical repair of congenital defects
Assessment of valvular function
Visualization
    Intracardiac air
    Atheroma (especially at the aortic cannulation site)
    Thrombi
    Myxomata
    Aortic dissection

*Complications*
Injury to airway/oesophagus
Bacteraemia
Distraction from direct patient care

The indications, uses and advantages of TOE are summarized in Table 2.4. Complications of TOE mainly relate to direct trauma to the airway and oesophagus and cardiac irritation from the probe resulting in atrial or ventricular dysrhythmias. TOE is contra-indicated in patients with known oesophageal pathology and because of the possibility of bacteraemia caused by instrumentation many clinicians feel that patients with prosthetic or abnormal valves should have standard antibiotic prophylaxis before TOE.

One serious indirect complication of intra-operative TOE is that the anaesthetist will be distracted from other aspects of patient care and monitoring whilst carrying out the echo study. Apart from exceptional circumstances, this is not a procedure to be undertaken by a lone, unassisted anaesthetist.

## Cerebral function monitoring

Significant, recognizable, neurological damage in the form of stroke occurs in 1–3% of patients following cardiopulmonary bypass. Neuropsychological complications are found in up to 70% (or more) of patients when carefully looked for. The majority of these deficits are minor and reversible but in the light of improving surgical mortality and morbidity efforts are being made to reduce the incidence of neurological problems. Patients vary in the degree to which they tolerate haemodynamic disturbances, and monitoring the electroencephalogram (EEG) gives some indication of the adequacy of cerebral function. Conventional EEG monitoring is cumbersome, and recording during surgery is difficult because of electrical interference. Interpretation is also difficult unless expert advice is available. Improvements in the display of information provided by an EEG have made cerebral function monitors more 'user-friendly'. The cerebral function analysing monitor (CFAM), for example, displays an upper trace made up of the maximum excursion, 90th centile, mean, 10th centile and minimum excursion of the processed EEG signal in each 2-sec epoch. Lower traces show the percentage of activity in each EEG waveband and the time the amplitude is depressed below 1.5 microvolts. Alternative approaches to analysis and display of EEG information include density-modulated spectral array technology and aperiodic analysis. In aperiodic analysis each wave of the EEG is converted to a vertical line whose height is proportional to the amplitude of the wave. Commercially available monitors display this information in an easily assimilated form with right and left cerebral hemispheres shown separately.

Despite improvements in EEG technology its use during cardiopulmonary bypass remains controversial. Individual studies (Nevin et al., 1989) have correlated EEG information with the prediction of neurological damage after bypass but many have shown no reasonable correlation between EEG abnormalities and neuropsychological outcome. It may be that although the EEG can demonstrate cerebral ischaemia produced by gross insults, such as unrecognized cerebrovascular stenoses or misplacement of the aortic cannula, it cannot reliably detect infarcts caused by small emboli. Cerebral function monitoring is, therefore, not yet considered sufficiently reliable or specific enough for use routinely during cardiopulmonary bypass and is not widely employed.

Potential alternatives to the CFAM device include transcranial Doppler (TCD) ultrasonography and near infra-red spectroscopy (NIRS). TCD may provide a useful non-invasive means of monitoring cerebral blood flow. During cardiopulmonary bypass (CPB) it has been used to measure blood flow in the middle cerebral artery, which is known to supply approximately 80% of the blood flow to the cerebrum. TCD has also been used to detect the passage of microemboli into the brain during CPB, although it is difficult to differentiate between air emboli and particulate matter. There is conflicting evidence, however, regarding the association between TCD-detected emboli and neurological dysfunction (Kahn, 1995). TCD devices are now available commercially, but this technique remains operator dependent and highly sensitive to movement artefact. TCD is a relatively accurate technique when used in the laboratory by a trained technician but is less user-friendly as a practical tool in the operating theatre.

Near infra-red spectroscopy (NIRS) is another method of monitoring cerebral blood flow and embolic events during CPB. NIRS is well established for studying cerebral oxygenation and haemodynamics in neonates using transmission spectroscopy, where light is shone across the whole head. In adults the thicker skull and larger head require a different technique of reflectance spectroscopy, with optodes placed a few centimetres apart on the same side of the head (Harris, 1995). NIRS appears to have many technical problems, including difficulty in accurate positioning of the optodes and differentiation between the intra- and extra-cranial circulation. It also samples a very small area of the cerebral blood supply and may not necessarily detect local hypoperfusion in 'watershed' areas during CPB. Hypothermic CPB, in particular, creates a number of problems because cooling and rewarming is uneven, cerebral oedema is produced and perfusion is abnormal even if pulsatile flow is used. In summary, NIRS has not yet been sufficiently refined or validated to be used as a monitor in the clinical setting during CPB.

## Induction of anaesthesia

After appropriate monitoring has been established and pre-oxygenation completed induction of anaesthesia is commenced. This is invariably achieved by the intravenous route in adults. The drugs used for induction will depend to some extent on what agents are to be used for maintenance. For example, if a high-dose opioid technique is to be employed then the chosen opioid (e.g. fentanyl) can be given slowly to provide sufficient depth of anaesthesia without significant depression of the myocardium. The addition of nitrous oxide to a high-dose opioid regime can, however, cause profound myocardial depression on rare occasions.

A more common approach to induction is to administer a moderate dose of opioid (fentanyl 5–10 µg per kg, alfentanil 50–100 µg per kg or remifentanil 1 µg per kg) before a minimal dose of etomidate, thiopentone or propofol, given by slow injection. This technique provides a smooth induction and minimizes the fall in arterial pressure, largely caused by a combination of myocardial depression and decrease in systemic vascular resistance when these latter agents are used alone in larger doses (Table 2.5).

Etomidate is currently our induction agent of choice for adult cardiac surgery. It has minimal effects on the cardiovascular system in normal subjects but does tend to decrease the arterial pressure in patients with cardiovascular disease, although to a lesser extent than other agents. Etomidate is, therefore, particularly useful when coronary perfusion is critical, for example, in patients with

**Table 2.5 Induction agents – cardiovascular effects**

|            | HR                              | SVR                   | CO        | Mean arterial BP |
|------------|---------------------------------|-----------------------|-----------|------------------|
| Thiopentone | Increase                       | Increase              | Decrease  | Decrease         |
| Etomidate  | Increase (slight)               | Decrease (slight)     | Unchanged | Unchanged        |
| Propofol   | Unchanged (or slight decrease)  | Decrease              | Decrease  | Decrease         |

HR, heart rate; SVR, systemic vascular resistance; CO, cardiac output; BP, blood pressure. Thiopentone: increase in heart rate and systemic vascular resistance are reflex changes. Propofol: cardiac output changes variable (see Bell *et al.*, 1995)

mainstem disease of the left coronary artery or aortic valve disease. Etomidate must be used with care in the elderly, however, in whom substantial falls in arterial pressure have been recorded following its use. In addition it is probable that etomidate causes some adrenal suppression even after a single dose.

Alternative techniques to those described above include the use of benzodiazepines and ketamine. Cardiovascular stability is well maintained when diazepam is used alone and therefore this drug can be used for sedation while invasive monitoring is established using local analgesia. Midazolam, the shorter acting benzodiazepine, can be used in this setting but it may decrease systemic vascular resistance at high dose levels or when used in combination with opioids. The substantial rise in arterial pressure associated with the use of ketamine is undesirable before the majority of cardiac surgery and the drug is little used for induction.

## Muscular relaxation

After induction of anaesthesia endotracheal intubation is carried out following the administration of a non-depolarizing muscle relaxant. Intermittent positive pressure ventilation (IPPV) can then be commenced.

Pancuronium (0.12–0.15 mg per kg) is widely used to provide muscular relaxation for cardiac surgery. This drug tends to cause a tachycardia and an elevation of arterial blood pressure caused by vagolytic and sympathomimetic actions (Table 2.6). These features were considered an advantage when pancuronium was first introduced before the expansion of cardiac surgery for

**Table 2.6 Muscle relaxants – cardiovascular effects**

|            | HR        | SVR                         | CO        | Mean arterial BP            |
|------------|-----------|-----------------------------|-----------|-----------------------------|
| Pancuronium | Increase  | Increase                    | Increase  | Increase                    |
| Vecuronium | Unchanged | Unchanged                   | Unchanged | Unchanged                   |
| Atracurium | Unchanged | Unchanged (or slight decrease) | Unchanged | Unchanged (or slight decrease) |

HR, heart rate; SVR, systemic vascular resistance; CO, cardiac output; BP, blood pressure. Pancuronium has marked vagolytic effect on the heart and sympathomimetic actions; rate can be controlled with beta-adrenergic blockade

coronary heart disease but could now be considered a disadvantage. In practice, however, a significant tachycardia is less likely in patients taking anti-anginal medication (particularly beta-adrenergic blocking agents) up to the time of surgery and the incidence of ischaemia associated with the use of pancuronium is very low if heart rate is pharmacologically controlled intra-operatively.

The shorter acting muscle relaxant vecuronium does not influence heart rate or arterial pressure in fit patients undergoing general anaesthesia and the newer agent rocuronium has a similar haemodynamic profile. Vecuronium should be considered for use in patients prone to tachy-dysrhythmias and those undergoing short procedures.

Atracurium does not seem to have a well-defined role in cardiac anaesthesia but may be used for short non-bypass procedures in patients who are cardiovascularly stable. A continuous infusion of atracurium is also used by some anaesthetists to facilitate early extubation following bypass surgery.

## Tracheal intubation

Tracheal intubation is normally secured via the oral route in adults undergoing routine cardiac surgery. Oral tubes are well tolerated in the early postoperative period. Nasal tubes are more likely to cause bleeding in the naso-pharynx following the administration of heparin and they may also pose an infection risk.

Double lumen endobronchial tubes are indicated for certain operations in adults such as repair of coarctation of the aorta or descending thoracic aneurysm.

This allows collapse of the lung on the operative (left) side to facilitate surgery. Where possible left-sided tubes are inserted to circumvent the problems associated with right upper lobe ventilation. Occasionally an adult will present for a modified Blalock shunt operation. This operation is designed to provide additional pulmonary blood flow via a synthetic tube graft inserted from the subclavian to pulmonary artery. One-lung anaesthesia can be useful in facilitating this type of surgery but must be employed with extreme care. Patients requiring palliative shunt surgery are always hypoxic and they may not tolerate one-lung anaesthesia. Misplacement of a double lumen tube in this situation can be catastrophic if unrecognized.

## Maintenance of anaesthesia

Anaesthesia not only provides complete analgesia and lack of awareness for the patient but also a means of promoting cardiovascular stability during the operative period. In the case of coronary artery disease systemic pressures are kept in the low–normal range, taking account of the pre-operative blood pressure and avoiding both tachycardia and hypertension in order to prevent myocardial ischaemia. Anaesthetic agents alone, however, can rarely provide complete haemodynamic control. Additional drug therapy with a variety of vasoactive drugs, including nitrates, vasoconstrictors and beta-adrenergic blocking agents, may also be required (see also Chapter 4)

An adequate depth of anaesthesia can be maintained with an inhalational agent alone or more commonly in combination with an intravenous opioid. Nitrous oxide should be used with care in patients with poor myocardial function because of its cardiodepressant effects which are more marked in combination with narcotics. Moffitt and Sethna (1986) have suggested that nitrous oxide should be avoided completely in patients with coronary disease because it 'involves an insidious risk of myocardial ischaemia not always identified by the ECG'. We now use an oxygen/air mix as the inspired gas and add to this a volatile inhalational agent. This approach also eliminates the possibility that nitrous oxide will enlarge micro air-emboli in the circulation post-bypass.

Morphine was originally used as the drug of choice for a high-dose opioid technique but this has been superseded by the shorter acting synthetic opioids. Fentanyl is probably the most commonly used opioid, but sufentanil (currently unavailable in the UK) is also popular. Alfentanil is also administered by some anaesthetists at induction, by infusion throughout surgery or as a bolus during the rewarming phase of bypass. Remifentanil, the new short-acting opioid, which is broken down by plasma and tissue esterases, is also being promoted for use by infusion during cardiac surgery.

Fentanyl has been used as a sole anaesthetic agent for cardiac surgery in doses as high as 50–100 µg per kg. Even at higher dose levels, however, fentanyl does not dependably abolish all autonomic stimulation and the decrease in circulating fentanyl levels at the onset of bypass is greater than can be attributed to dilution alone. This is probably because fentanyl (unlike alfentanil) is taken up by the membrane oxgenator. The elimination half-life of fentanyl is, on the other hand, prolonged in the post-bypass period. The majority of anaesthetists therefore now use fentanyl in more moderate doses (10–30 µg per kg), in combination with a suitable inhalational agent, and take further steps to prevent awareness during the bypass period. This latter technique is more suitable when early tracheal extubation is planned.

Cardiovascular effects of the inhalational agents isoflurane, enflurane and halothane are summarized in Table 2.7. The newer agents desflurane and sevoflurane, which provide a rapid uptake and recovery, are less likely to be used intra-operatively during relatively long cardiac procedures. Sevoflurane is, however, a suitable induction agent for children with cardiac disease.

Isoflurane was initially heralded as the ideal cardiac anaesthetic agent because it preserved cardiac output with a reduced peripheral resistance and did not significantly depress myocardial contractility. Subsequent studies focused attention on the coronary vasodilator effect of isoflurane, however. These studies showed that, in certain circumstances, isoflurane can cause a deleterious

**Table 2.7 Inhalational agents – cardiovascular effects**

|  | HR | SVR | CO | Mean arterial BP |
|---|---|---|---|---|
| Enflurane | Increase | Decrease | Decrease | Decrease |
| Halothane | Unchanged | Decrease | Decrease | Decrease |
| Isoflurane | Increase | Decrease | Maintained | Decrease |

HR, heart rate; SVR, systemic vascular resistance; CO, cardiac output; BP, blood pressure. Of the above agents, isoflurane has the least depressant effect on myocardial function/contractility

redistribution of coronary blood flow. Thus isoflurane can increase blood flow to healthy areas of myocardium by diverting it from potentially ischaemic areas supplied by diseased coronary arteries; the so-called 'coronary steal' effect. The prevalence of patients prone to coronary steal has been investigated by Buffington *et al.* (1988). In a retrospective study based on the Coronary Artery Surgery Study (CASS) this group estimated that 23% of the patients had 'steal-prone' coronary anatomy.

The controversy surrounding use of isoflurane has overshadowed interest in the other agents, halothane and enflurane. The classic work of Moffit and Sethna (1986) has shown that the combination of an opioid such as fentanyl with halothane or enflurane as the potent inhalational agent provides near ideal anaesthesia for the patient with good ventricular function. In their studies both agents caused controlled myocardial depression but myocardial oxygen consumption was also reduced to a greater degree so that myocardial oxygen supply was not compromised and myocardial ischaemia was not a feature of their use. Halothane and enflurane therefore remain a sensible choice of anaesthetic agent for cardiac surgery in patients with good ventricular function.

Despite this evidence, briefly discussed above, other work tends to suggest that the choice of anaesthetic agent does not significantly affect the outcome of coronary artery surgery (Slogoff and Keats, 1989; Tuman *et al.*, 1989b).

In practice isoflurane is widely used during cardiac surgery but in relatively low doses, which are less likely to cause a 'steal' phenomenon, and in combination with an opioid. In addition isoflurane is less likely to sensitize the myocardium to catecholamines and is therefore useful in the presence of significant cardiac arrhythmias. Isoflurane is also the volatile agent of choice (of the older longer acting drugs) if there is the possibility of halogen-induced hepatitis after repeat exposure to anaesthetic agents. Recent evidence (Ebert *et al.*, 1997) suggests that the use of sevoflurane results in a similar incidence of cardiac complications as isoflurane, in adults with cardiac disease having non-cardiac surgery. Sevoflurane is, at present, substantially more expensive than isoflurane, however.

In addition to the combination of opioid drugs and inhalational agents described above many anaesthetists use intravenous benzodiazepines during surgery to prevent awareness. The shorter acting drug midazolam is commonly used and this may be given at induction, just before cardiopulmonary bypass is commenced and during the rewarming phase of bypass. We tend to restrict the use of benzodiazepines to longer more complex cases where we do not plan to extubate the patient early.

Alternative approaches to anaesthesia during the period of cardiopulmonary bypass include the administration of volatile agents via the oxygenator and the use of a propofol infusion. We use isoflurane administered via a separate vaporizer on the bypass machine but it is difficult to judge the dose levels necessary to prevent awareness. In addition it is possible that the concentration of the agent will be turned down by the perfusionist when vascular resistance is low. It is helpful to monitor the concentration of isoflurane escaping from the exhaust port of the oxygenator so that everyone concerned has a reasonable idea of the inspired concentration and can therefore act accordingly. Isoflurane 2% has been shown to reduce significantly the cortisol response during bypass, albeit combined with a large dose of fentanyl given at the start of surgery. Isoflurane at 1% also attenuates cortisol levels, but to a lesser extent.

Propofol, the short-acting induction agent, has been used by infusion either alone or in combination with an opioid to provide anaesthesia during cardiac surgery. The main cardiovascular effect of this drug is hypotension, caused by a combination of vasodilatation and mild myocardial depression. It is not a suitable induction agent for all patients (for example those with poor ventricular function, the elderly and those patients with aortic stenosis) but it can be used intra-operatively, with care, in the majority of patients. Propofol with its short duration of action, lack of accumulation and profound venodilator effect is particularly useful to provide anaesthesia by infusion during cardiopulmonary bypass once an adequate perfusion pressure has been established. A rigid dose regime has not been established but it appears that relatively low infusion rates (4 mg per kg per hour) can be used to provide hypnosis and amnesia during cardiopulmonary bypass when the drug is used in combination with moderate doses of fentanyl. The target controlled infusion (TCI) system can also be adapted for use during cardiac surgery and propofol may be continued in to the postoperative period in order to facilitate early awakening and extubation of suitable patients.

## Summary

This chapter has provided a broad overview of anaesthetic techniques used during adult cardiac surgery. The development of cardiac anaesthesia has been an evolutionary process. A few older references are therefore provided along side more recent review articles, following this chapter, so that the reader may appreciate this process.

The intra-operative management of specific cardiac and allied operations are described in more detail in the next chapter.

## References

Bell J., Sartain J., Wilkinson G.A.L. and Sherry K.M. (1995) Comparison of propofol and fentanyl anaesthesia in coronary artery versus valve surgery. *Anaesthesia;* **50:** 644–648.

Buffington C.W., Davis K.B., Gillespie S. and Pettinger M. (1988) The prevalence of steal-prone anatomy in patients with coronary artery disease: an analysis of the Coronary Artery Surgery Study registry. *Anesthesiology;* **69:** 721–727.

Ebert T.J., Kharasch E.V., Rooke G.A. *et al.* (1997) Myocardial ischaemia and adverse cardiac outcome in cardiac patients undergoing noncardiac surgery with sevoflurane and isoflurane. *Anesth Analg;* **85:** 993–999.

English I.C.W., Frew R.M., Pigott J.F. and Zaki M. (1969) Percutaneous catheterization of the internal jugular vein. *Anaesthesia;* **24:** 521–526.

Harris D.N.F. (1995) Near infra-red spectroscopy. Editorial. *Anaesthesia;* **50:** 1015–1016.

Kahn R.A., Slogoff F.A., Reich D.L. and Konstadt S.N. (1995) Transcranial Doppler ultra-sonography: what is its role in cardiac and vascular surgical patients? *J Cardiothorac Vasc Anesth;* **9:** 589–597.

Liban B.J. and Davies D.M. (1986) Elective coronary bypass surgery without pulmonary artery catheter monitoring. *Anesthesiology;* **64:** 664–665.

Moffit E.A. and Sethna D.H. (1986) The coronary circulation and myocardial oxygenation in coronary artery disease: effects of anesthesia. *Anesth Analg;* **65:** 395–410.

Nevin M., Colchester A.C.F., Adams S. and Pepper J.R. (1989) Prediction of neurological damage after cardiopulmonary bypass surgery. *Anaesthesia;* **44:** 725–729.

Reves J.G., Sladen R.N. and Newman M.F. (1995) Cardiac anesthetic: is it unique? *Anesth Analg;* **81:** 895–896.

Slogoff S. and Keats A.S. (1989) Randomized trial of primary anesthetic agents on outcome of coronary bypass operations. *Anesthesiology;* **70:** 179–188.

Tuman K.J., McCarthy R.J., Speiss B.D. *et al.* (1989a) Effect of pulmonary artery catheterization on outcome in patients undergoing coronary artery surgery. *Anesthesiology;* **70:** 432–437.

Tuman K.J, McCarthy R.J., Spiess B.D. *et al.* (1989b) Does choice of anesthetic agent significantly effect outcome after coronary artery surgery? *Anesthesiology;* **70:** 189–198.

# Chapter 3

# Anaesthesia for specific cardiac and allied operations

## Coronary artery surgery

Coronary artery disease is the leading cause of death in developed countries; thus it is not surprising that coronary artery bypass grafting represents the bulk of cardiac surgery performed worldwide. This procedure ranges from low-risk elective surgery, with a mortality of less than 1%, to very high-risk surgery in patients presenting as an emergency with poor ventricular function or significant co-morbid disease.

It is important that the anaesthetist should make some assessment of the severity of the coronary artery disease prior to surgery so that the risk of intra-operative myocardial ischaemia may be quantified. The reader is referred to Chapter 1 for details of the pre-operative assessment of the patient with ischaemic heart disease.

Angiographic factors indicating an increased risk of peri-operative ischaemia include:

- Left main stem disease: the left coronary artery divides to form the left anterior descending and the circumflex arteries, which in turn supply the majority of the left ventricle and interventricular septum
- Proximal left anterior descending and circumflex lesions: this amounts to a left main stem equivalent combination
- Poor distal vessels: if the distal coronary arteries are small, or have diffuse disease, even following revascularization the flow of blood through the vessels will be low predisposing to early graft occlusion.

Prevention of peri-operative ischaemia is dependent upon the optimization of myocardial oxygen supply and demand. The majority of patients presenting for coronary artery bypass grafting are already receiving drugs with this aim in mind. These include beta-blockers, which reduce the heart rate thus reducing myocardial oxygen demand. Beta-blockers also increase diastolic perfusion time and improve subendocardial blood flow by controlling hypertension, thus increasing the myocardial oxygen supply. Calcium channel antagonists and nitrates may also be used to promote coronary vasodilatation, again increasing myocardial oxygen supply in the presence of coronary artery disease. These drugs must be given on the morning of surgery as abrupt withdrawal may result in rebound hypertension, tachycardia and loss of coronary vasodilatation at a critical time.

## Anaesthetic management

Although intra-operative ischaemia is not always directly the result of adverse haemodynamic changes, some certainly is, and therefore attention must be paid to avoiding undesirable swings in heart rate and blood pressure. Thus, adequate premedication prior to coronary artery bypass surgery is essential to minimize tachycardia and hypertension. In our institution temazepam is commonly used for premedication. It is occasionally necessary, in particularly anxious patients, to supplement this with a small dose of an intravenous benzodiazepine such as midazolam, prior to invasive monitoring line insertion.

After vascular access has been gained, an arterial monitoring line is placed. ECG leads and a pulse oximetry probe are sited and induction of anaesthesia is commenced with the principal aim of avoiding extremes of blood pressure and heart rate. We use a high-dose opioid technique in order achieve this aim, further details of which may be found in Chapter 2. It is common following tracheal intubation, whilst central venous access is being gained, for the blood pressure to gradually decrease. The pre-induction insertion of an arterial monitoring line allows the rapid detection and treatment of hypotension. If ventricular function is known to be good, hypotension may be corrected with the infusion of intravenous fluids. If, however, the hypotension is severe, or the ventricular function is compromised, it is preferable to administer an alpha receptor agonist such as phenylephrine to restore the diastolic pressure, and therefore coronary perfusion. Metaraminol, although commonly used in this situation, is less desirable as it is a mixed alpha- and beta receptor agonist. It may therefore also increase heart rate and myocardial contractility, resulting in an increase in myocardial oxygen demand and reduced coronary perfusion time.

Other events during the course of surgery, which are associated with major haemodynamic changes and therefore may predispose to ischaemia, include sternotomy, sternal retraction for internal mammary artery dissection, and pericardial and aortic dissection. It is important to have intravenous fluids and drugs such as glyceryl trinitrate, fentanyl and phenylephrine immediately available in order to attenuate these responses.

It must be remembered that myocardial ischaemia is also common post-bypass despite adequate revascularization. This may be due to coronary artery spasm, or spasm in arterial or even saphenous vein grafts. Spasm appears to be particularly associated with radial arterial grafts, it is therefore advisable to continue an infusion of a vasodilator drug such as glyceryl trinitrate well into the postoperative period. In the case of radial arterial grafts many surgeons also routinely use calcium antagonists in order promote postoperative graft dilatation.

# Minimally invasive cardiac surgery

In recent years there has been a huge development in minimally invasive surgical techniques. These are popular with patients as they result in smaller scars, and popular with hospital managers as they result in a shorter duration of hospital stay and therefore may reduce costs. The advent of minimally invasive cardiac surgery was rather delayed relative to other specialities as cross-clamping the aorta and providing adequate myocardial protection was difficult to achieve via an endoscope or minithoracotomy incision. This problem was solved in two ways; firstly the definition of minimally invasive was expanded to include not only surgery via small incisions, but also cardiac surgery performed without the 'invasion' of cardiopulmonary bypass. Thus minimally invasive cardiac surgery is now divided into that performed via small incisions or ports utilizing bypass, and that performed through a variety of incisions including median sternotomy on the beating heart, without the use of cardiopulmonary bypass.

## Minimally invasive cardiac surgery with cardiopulmonary bypass

The development of a novel balloon tipped endoaortic clamp (Fig. 3.1) has recently enabled cardiopulmonary bypass to be instituted via the femoral vessels, the aorta to be occluded by an intraortic balloon and cardioplegia to be delivered via the endoaortic clamp into the aortic root, all without opening the thoracic cavity. This technique has been used for anterior coronary artery bypass grafts, mitral valve repair and replacement and more recently, aortic valve replacement.

## Anaesthetic management

In addition to the usual anaesthetic management of patients undergoing cardiac surgery (see Chapter 2), a left-sided double lumen endobronchial tube is inserted and its position confirmed with fibre-optic bronchoscopy. Bilateral radial arterial lines are sited and, in addition to a quadruple lumen catheter, a 9-French sheath is also placed in the right internal jugular vein. If mitral valve surgery is planned

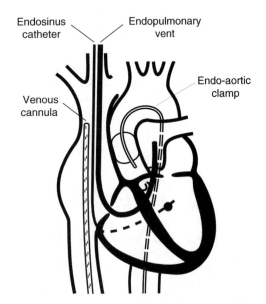

**Fig. 3.1** Novel catheters used in minimally invasive cardiac surgery with cardiopulmonary bypass

a second 10-French sheath may also be sited in a central vein. The transoesophageal echocardiography probe is inserted following the induction of anaesthesia.

## Conduct of surgery

In the case of coronary artery bypass grafting, a small left anterior thoracotomy incision is made to allow dissection of the internal mammary artery, either under direct vision or with thoracoscopic assistance. Visualization may be assisted by the use of a double lumen endobronchial tube enabling one lung ventilation during this period of the surgery. Heparin, 300 units/kg, is then given and the arterial and venous cannulae are inserted into the femoral vessels. The venous cannula is passed under fluoroscopic control, over a guidewire into the superior vena cava. The endoaortic clamp is advanced via the arterial cannula so that its tip lies in the ascending aorta, approximately 2–4 cm from the aortic valve. An 8.3-French single lumen endopulmonary vent is simultaneously railroaded over a pulmonary artery catheter by the anaesthetist to lie in the main pulmonary artery. This drains via an air relief valve into the cardiopulmonary bypass venting line, thus allowing venting of the heart during bypass. The endopulmonary vent may also significantly contribute to the venous return. Cardiopulmonary bypass is then commenced, the lumen of the ascending aorta is occluded by the inflation of the balloon surrounding the tip of the endoaortic clamp and then cardioplegia is infused into the aortic root via a central lumen. The surgery may then be carried out on an arrested heart via the anterior thoracotomy.

The success of this system is critically dependent upon stable and effective occlusion of the aorta by the endoclamp. If the balloon drifts into the aortic root it may damage the aortic valve or even become displaced into the left ventricle. If it moves into the aortic arch it may obstruct the innominate artery which subsequently gives rise to the right internal carotid artery, thus significantly impairing cerebral perfusion. The position of the endoclamp balloon is therefore constantly monitored with transoesophageal echocardiograpy. Distal movement is also readily detected by the use of bilateral radial arterial monitoring lines. If the innominate artery becomes occluded it will be revealed as a decrease in right radial arterial pressure relative to the left. Another factor to consider is that in order to achieve a stable position, with effective occlusion of the ascending aorta, an unphysiologically high pressure must be generated within the balloon (250–350 mmHg). It is not yet known whether this is associated with significant aortic injury, particularly in the presence of atheromatous plaques in the aorta. It is, however, known that conventional clamping may cause aortic dissection under these circumstances and balloon clamping may be a useful alternative approach (Falk *et al.,* 1996).

Further haemodynamic monitoring used includes the aortic root pressure, pulmonary artery pressure, balloon pressure and central venous pressure. Pulsed wave Doppler of the right carotid artery may also be used to detect distal migration of the endoaortic clamp. When the surgery is complete the balloon is deflated and the endoclamp is withdrawn via the femoral arterial cannula. Pacing wires may be sited via the minithoracotomy incision, and the heart defibrillated with paediatric defibrillation paddles if necessary. Bypass is discontinued when appropriate (see Chapter 4) and the heparin neutralized with protamine in the usual manner.

During mitral valve surgery, an additional coronary sinus catheter may be sited under fluoroscopic and echocardiographic control in order to allow the delivery of retrograde cardioplegia.

The disadvantages of the above technique are that the need for cardiopulmonary bypass is not eliminated, and that the procedure is generally relatively prolonged as the accurate siting of the various cannulae is time consuming.

The advantages, however, include the fact that this technique appears to be applicable to valve surgery as well as coronary artery surgery. Also the patient does not undergo median sternotomy and therefore the incidence of wound infection and sternal breakdown is reduced. Recovery is fast and the duration of hospital stay is potentially shorter. The intensity of early postoperative pain is, however, much greater that that associated with a median sternotomy, and achieving an adequate level of analgesia may be difficult. We have found that the combination of a morphine infusion, diclofenac (if there are no contraindications) and intercostal blocks is effective in these patients.

## Minimally invasive cardiac surgery without cardiopulmonary bypass

Minimally invasive direct vision coronary artery bypass surgery (MIDCAB) may be performed via a median sternotomy, minithoracotomy or parasternal incision upon a beating heart, thus avoiding all the problems associated with cardiopulmonary bypass. This technique was originally introduced in the treatment of solitary lesions of the left anterior descending artery; it may now, with the development of improved mechanical stabilizing devices, be extended to patients with more extensive disease.

### Anaesthetic management

The induction of anaesthesia for MIDCAB surgery should promote a slow stable heart rate. Thus pancuronium should be avoided and careful attention paid to the adequacy of the depth of anaesthesia. Following induction, if a minithoracotomy approach is planned, a double lumen endobronchial tube is inserted. One lung ventilation may then be used to aid visualization during internal mammary artery harvest and also to minimize myocardial movement due to ventilation during the performance of the anastomosis. If a median sternotomy is used, a single lumen endotracheal tube is adequate; excessive myocardial movement associated with ventilation may then be minimized by reducing the rate, tidal volume or both.

The force and rate of cardiac contraction greatly affects the ease of the surgical anastomosis; this can be modulated either by pharmacological or mechanical manoeuvres.

### Pharmacological manipulation of heart rate

A short-acting beta-blocker such as esmolol may be used to reduce the heart rate and provide a 'quieter field' in which the anastomosis can be performed. Heart rates between 40 and 60 beats/min may be readily achieved with an infusion of 50–200 mcg/kg/min. This bradycardia may be rapidly reversed by stopping the infusion or by the stimulation of the heart by the surgeon. If a more profound bradycardia or even a period of brief cardiac standstill is required, adenosine 3–12 mg may also be given. This drug delays conduction through the atrioventricular node and as its half-life is only 10 sec it must be given by rapid intravenous injection. It must be remembered that although the effects of adenosine may be reversed by theophylline or caffeine, they are not by atropine.

As the reduction in heart rate is generally accompanied by a decrease in systemic blood pressure a vasoconstrictor such as phenylephrine should be used to maintain coronary perfusion. This can be given in increments of 50 mcg, or perhaps more satisfactorily by intravenous infusion. Glyceryl trinitrate must be given throughout the procedure in order to promote coronary vasodilatation.

### Mechanical manipulation of the surgical field

As an alternative to the pharmacological control of the heart rate, which may on occasion be unpredictable, various devices are under investigation which act to mechanically restrain the surgical field. One such device, the Utrecht Octopus, is applied to the heart via suction cups and acts by restraining a relatively small $3 \times 4$ cm part of the ventricle. The heart is then lifted by the device into a position optimum for surgery (Grundeman et al., 1997). This displacement of the heart is often associated with a fall in cardiac output, which may be attenuated by volume loading prior to cardiac displacement and placing the patient in the Trendelenberg position.

A reduced dose of heparin 100 units/kg is given prior to the anastomoses. These patients also receive beta-blocking drugs, either prior to surgery or following induction of anaesthesia in order to further optimize surgical conditions. It is essential that cardiopulmonary bypass is 'standing by' as severe haemodynamic instability may occur following cardiac displacement.

Although the MIDCAB technique seems attractive, it is possible, that the benefits associated with avoiding bypass are gained at the expense of the quality of the surgery, it is significantly more difficult to perform a good anastomosis on a beating heart. Certainly, preliminary reports do suggest an increased graft occlusion rate in patients undergoing this procedure.

### Minimally invasive long saphenous vein harvest

The minimally invasive approach to cardiac surgery has also been extended to the long saphenous vein harvest. Multiple 3–4 cm incisions along the course of the vein have been shown to reduce postoperative pain and improve healing thus facilitating early mobilization (Tevaearai et al., 1997). The risk of conduit damage, however, may be increased and this technique has not yet gained widespread support.

## Transmyocardial laser revascularization

The mainstay of treatment of ischaemic heart disease is currently coronary revascularization, either by coronary artery bypass grafting or angioplasty. However, there is an increasing population of patients who suffer from debilitating angina, but are not suitable for treatment with either of these techniques. These patients may benefit from transmyocardial laser revascularization (TMR). This is a newly developed technique that aims to improve myocardial blood flow and reduce anginal symptoms.

During TMR a high energy, 850 watt laser is applied to the ischaemic area in order to create between 15 and 60 transmyocardial channels. The assumption is that these channels, once formed remain patent, providing direct perfusion of the myocardium with ventricular blood. This is analogous to the mechanism underlying reptilian myocardial perfusion, and certainly in some studies it has been shown that the channels are still patent 30 days after the laser treatment, supporting the theory that blood must be flowing through them (Horvath *et al.*, 1996). Although this theory is attractive, the mechanism of action may be more complex. It may also be postulated that the inflammation associated with production of the channels may lead to neovascularization of the surrounding area of myocardium, thus improving its blood supply. Alternatively, the channels created may simply undergo fibrous scarring, thus reducing the myocardial oxygen demand of that region of the ventricle and resulting in a reduction in the severity of the angina.

**Table 3.1 Indications for transmyocardial laser revascularization**

Primary therapy when a contraindication to cardiopulmonary bypass exists

Absence of suitable conduit

Severe coronary artery disease not amenable to coronary artery bypass grafting or percutaneous transluminal coronary angioplasty

Severe coronary artery disease following heart transplantation

Angina refractory to medical therapy

Unacceptable side effects of medical therapy

The indications for TMR are shown in Table 3.1. These patients undergo extensive pre-operative evaluation in order to confirm their suitability for the technique. In addition to the general investigations that would be carried out on any patient undergoing cardiac surgery (see Chapter 1), a gamut of specialized cardiological tests is also performed. This assessment is primarily concerned with the evaluation of the size and the degree of reversibility of the ischaemic area (Table 3.2). By the nature of the indications for TMR, the patients selected for this procedure tend to have co-morbid disease such as hypertension, diabetes, chronic obstructive pulmonary disease and peripheral vascular disease. They may have impaired ventricular function, they will certainly have severe myocardial ischaemia, and are likely to have undergone previous cardiac surgery. These factors all indicate that anaesthesia and surgery constitute a significant risk to these patients.

## Anaesthesia for transmyocardial laser revascularization

Prior to induction, venous and arterial access should be gained. Anaesthesia is then induced and a left-sided double lumen tube inserted. As the surgery is

**Table 3.2 Investigations prior to transmyocardial laser revascularization**

| Investigation | Aim |
| --- | --- |
| Coronary angiography | Evaluation of coronary artery anatomy |
| Echocardiography | Evaluation of regional ventricular wall motion abnormalities and valvular function |
| Thallium-201 single photon emission computed tomography ($^{201}$TI-SPECT) | Evaluation of myocardial perfusion |
| Positron emission tomography (PET) | Evaluation of myocardial ischaemia and viability |
| Multigrade acquisition radionuclide ventriculography (MUGA) | Evaluation of left ventricular ejection fraction at rest |
| Dobutamine stress echocardiography or magnetic resonance imaging (MRI) | Evaluation of regional ventricular wall abnormalities and rest and on exercise |

generally via a left anterior thoracotomy incision, the double lumen tube aids surgical access by allowing deflation of the left lung. If one lung ventilation is employed, particular care should be taken to ensure that adequate ventilation and oxygenation are maintained. Hypoxia and hypercarbia in the presence of severe ischaemic heart disease may rapidly lead to arrhythmias and hypotension.

If not already secured, central venous access should be gained with a quadruple lumen catheter and a pulmonary artery catheter. An epidural catheter, transoesophageal echocardiography probe and external defibrillator pads are sited. The patient's eyes are protected and covered with damp gauze. Once transfer into theatre is complete the patient is carefully positioned with a sandbag under the left chest, taking care to prevent traction on the brachial plexus. A second set of ECG electrodes is applied to the patient and connected to the laser. This allows synchronization of the laser beam with the R wave of the cardiac cycle, thus reducing the risk of arrhythmias. The laser is then applied to the ischaemic myocardium, each pulse lasting 30–50 msec. An echo dense 'puff' of vaporized blood detected by the transoesophageal echocardiograph confirms that the channel created has extended throughout the full thickness of the myocardium (Fig. 3.2). Occasionally it may be necessary for a suture to be applied to the epicardium to prevent excessive bleeding from the created channels.

Inotropic drugs should not be used if at all possible during this procedure. The benefits of TMR are not effective immediately and an increase in myocardial oxygen consumption at this stage must be avoided. Normothermia is maintained and an infusion of glyceryl trinitrate may be beneficial. Nitrous oxide is not used as there is a theoretical risk that the microbubbles created by vaporizing the blood may be enlarged in its presence and predispose to gas embolus.

Postoperatively the patient is nursed in the intensive care unit. Analgesia is provided by the infusion of an opioid and a local anaesthetic agent via the epidural catheter. It should be remembered that the pain associated with a thoracotomy incision is potentially much greater than that of the sternotomy that the patient is likely to have experienced before. Ineffective analgesia may

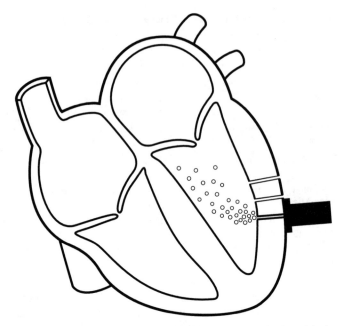

**Fig. 3.2** Schematic representation of  transmyocardial laser revascularization of the heart

therefore provoke anxiety. This coupled with tachycardia and hypertension is highly undesirable in the early postoperative period.

### Outcome following transmyocardial laser resection

Following TMR there appears to be an immediate subjective reduction in symptoms. This is probably a placebo effect. However at 3–6 months postoperatively, there is an average reduction in angina of two classes and improved regional blood flow has been demonstrated with positron emission tomography (Frazier *et al.,* 1995).

Thus although transmyocardial laser resection is a developing technique and its mechanism of action is not yet fully understood, it may prove to be a useful option in a high-risk group of patients in whom alternative treatment options are limited.

## Valvular surgery

### Aortic valve surgery

In the management of patients with valvular heart disease, the control of heart rate, preload and afterload in the prebypass period become particularly important (Table 3.3). In the presence of aortic incompetence, a heart rate slightly higher than usual at 80–100 beats/min combined with the use of vasodilators to produce a low systemic vascular resistance will reduce ventricular distension, the size of the regurgitant fraction, and also improve subendocardial blood flow.

**Table 3.3 Haemodynamic management prior to cardiopulmonary bypass in valvular heart disease**

|  | Heart rate | Preload | Afterload |
| --- | --- | --- | --- |
| Aortic stenosis | 60–80 beats/min maintain sinus rhythm | Upper end of normal range | Avoid reduction |
| Aortic incompetence | 80–100 beats/min | Normal range | Reduce SVR Avoid diastolic hypotension |
| Mitral stenosis | 60–80 beats/min Avoid atrial fibrillation | Upper end of normal range | Normal range Avoid increases in PVR |
| Mitral incompetence | 80–100 beats/min | Normal range | Avoid increases in SVR |

(Subendocardial perfusion pressure = aortic pressure – left ventricular pressure).

Conversely, if the aortic valve is stenotic a heart rate of 60–80 beats/min is appropriate to maintain the cardiac output. The blood pressure and systemic vascular resistance must be maintained within the normal range to preserve coronary filling. Although moderately raised filling pressures may be necessary to maintain the cardiac output, excessive infusion of intravenous fluids should be avoided as this predisposes to a rise in the left ventricular end diastolic pressure and consequently a fall in subendocardial perfusion. The loss of sinus rhythm in the presence of aortic stenosis may have a disastrous effect on ventricular filling and must be treated rapidly and effectively.

## Mitral valve surgery

As with aortic regurgitation, in mitral regurgitation the heart rate should be maintained between 80 and 100 beats/min. Most patients with long-standing mitral incompetence have atrial fibrillation, this results in a loss of the atrial 'kick' to ventricular filling and therefore a higher heart rate is necessary to maintain the cardiac output. Increases in systemic vascular resistance must be avoided in order to decrease the regurgitant fraction and maintain the cardiac output.

Conversely, in the presence of mitral stenosis the heart rate should be maintained within the normal range. Both reductions in left atrial pressure (i.e. preload) and a bradycardia or tachycardia will considerably reduce left ventricular filling. Thus the onset of atrial fibrillation in the presence of mitral stenosis may be associated with a sudden severe fall in cardiac output and the associated ventricular rate must be rapidly brought under control. Mitral stenosis may also eventually be complicated by pulmonary hypertension. The increase in pulmonary vascular resistance will reduce left atrial filling and also ultimately lead to right ventricular failure. Factors such as hypercarbia, hypoxia and acidosis will further increase the pulmonary vascular resistance and must be avoided. Similarly nitrous oxide, which is known to increase pulmonary vascular resistance, should not be used in the presence of pulmonary hypertension.

### Tricuspid valve

Disease of the tricuspid valve is less common than that of the aortic or mitral valves. Tricuspid regurgitation is usually due to right heart dilatation secondary to pulmonary hypertension and mitral valve disease. Generally the nature of the associated mitral valve disease and the severity of the pulmonary hypertension should dictate the anaesthetic management, rather than the tricuspid valve disease itself, which is often entirely asymptomatic. Careful fluid management, however, is essential, as in the presence of a dilated right ventricle hypovolaemia may result in a dramatic decrease in cardiac output. Conversely, overtransfusion may result in further compromise of ventricular function. Unfortunately the right atrial pressure is a poor indicator of volaemic status in the presence of tricuspid regurgitation, as the atrium and vena cavae are very compliant and a large change in volume may not be associated with any change in the recorded pressure. Transoesophageal echocardiography is a useful monitor in this situation.

Tricuspid stenosis or atresia is a rare congenital abnormality of the heart and as such its discussion is beyond the scope of this book.

Following any intracardiac operation any air present in the cardiac chambers must be evacuated before the heart is allowed to eject. This may be achieved by manipulation of the heart and aspiration with a needle and syringe. Air may be displaced into the left atrium (from which it may be aspirated) from the pulmonary veins by manually ventilating the patient. Transoesophageal echo-cardiography is useful tool to detect the presence of intracardiac air, thus facilitating its removal. Sites where air commonly collects include the left atrial appendage, the interatrial septum and the pulmonary veins. Following weaning from cardiopulmonary bypass the TOE is also useful in assessing the adequacy of valve repair, prosthetic valve function and diagnosing the presence of paraprosthetic leaks. In the presence of long-standing valvular heart disease, it is likely that ventricular function may be impaired and inotropes may be necessary in the early postoperative period. This topic is dealt with in greater detail in Chapter 5.

### Grown-up congenital heart disease

Many patients with complex congenital heart disease now survive to adulthood. In the USA there are over 600 000 surviving patients with congenital heart disease, the majority of whom have undergone some form of corrective or palliative surgery. In the UK there are approximately 200 operations carried out for grown-up congenital heart (GUCH) disease per annum and these figures are likely to increase. First-time cardiac operations are carried out because the malfunction was not detected earlier or because it was not considered severe enough to warrant surgery during childhood. Re-operations are more common for GUCH disease, however. In this latter category some patients require a definitive repair following previous corrective surgery. This includes replacement of valves and right-sided conduits, or repair of residual septal defects.

Our experience of surgery for adult congenital heart disease, from 1991–1994, is summarized in Tables 3.4 and 3.5 (Dore et al., 1997). First-time surgery for

**Table 3.4 First operations for 128 adults with congenital heart disease in Royal Brompton Hospital (UK) 1991–94**

| Type of surgery | Number of operations | Number of deaths |
| --- | --- | --- |
| Corrective repair | 123 | 5 |
| ASD | 40 | 0 |
| AVR | 31 | 0 |
| Coarctation of aorta | 14 | 0 |
| VSD | 9 | 0 |
| Tetralogy of Fallot | 4 | 1 |
| Fontan-type surgery | 3 | 1 |
| Other surgery | 22 | 3 |
| Palliative repair | 5 | 0 |
| Modified Blalock shunt* | 5 | 0 |

*Modified Blalock shunt, i.e. systemic arterial to pulmonary artery shunt. ASD, atrial septal defect; AVR, aortic valve replacement; VSD, ventricular septal defect
Adapted from Dore *et al.*, 1997

**Table 3.5 Re-operations for 167 adults (179 procedures) with congenital heart disease. Royal Brompton Hospital (UK) 1991–1994**

| Type of surgery | Number of operations | Number of deaths |
| --- | --- | --- |
| Corrective repair | 49 | 5 |
| AVR | 17 | 0 |
| Tetralogy of Fallot | 7 | 1 |
| Fontan-type surgery | 5 | 0 |
| Repair of DORV | 3 | 3 |
| Other surgery | 17 | 1 |
| Re-operations after corrective repair | 115 | 10 |
| AVR | 43 | 4 |
| Change of conduit | 30 | 4 |
| Re-coarctation of aorta | 11 | 1 |
| Other surgery | 31 | 1 |
| Further palliation | 15 | 1 |
| Modified Blalock shunt | 12 | 1 |
| Glenn shunt | 3 | 0 |

DORV, double outlet right ventricle
Adapted from *Dore et al.*, 1997

aortic valve replacement and closure of atrial septal defect carried no mortality in our series. This is not surprising in patients with preserved myocardial function and few of the sequelae of chronic heart disease. Mortality is higher in surgery for repair of tetralogy of Fallot and Fontan-type surgery, however, where pre-operative cyanosis and myocardial dysfunction are particularly relevant.

Re-operations (179 of 307 operations) were carried out in a greater number of patients than first-time surgery. For corrective repair mortality was acceptable at 10.2% (Table 3.5), with the exception of repair of double outlet right ventricle in which there were 3 deaths from 3 operations. Re-operations after previous corrective surgery carried a mortality of 8.7%, but the mortality relating to conduit change was significantly higher than this at 13.3% (4 deaths from 30 operations).

The detailed management of individual forms of GUCH disease is beyond the scope of this book. There have, however, been several extensive reviews on this topic to which the interested reader is referred (Baum, 1996; Baum and Perloff, 1993; Findlow and Doyle, 1997). The main risk factors in GUCH patients presenting for surgery are, however, discussed below, together with the principles of anaesthetic and peri-operative management.

## Risk factors

The major risk factors for mortality and morbidity in GUCH patients presenting for anaesthesia and cardiac surgery are:

● Increased pulmonary vascular resistance
● Chronic cyanosis
● Abnormal renal function
● Ventricular dysfunction
● Dysrhythmias
● Problems associated with re-operation.

### Increased pulmonary vascular resistance

Patients are unlikely to be referred for corrective cardiac surgery if they are known to have significant pulmonary hypertension. A fixed pulmonary arteriolar resistance index above normal levels is, for example an absolute contra-indication to any form of right heart bypass procedure such as the modified Fontan operation (Hosking and Beynen, 1992). In patients with severe pulmonary stenosis, however, it may be difficult to accurately measure pressure in the pulmonary arteries. It is unlikely, if this is the case, that these patients will have developed pulmonary hypertension unless there are large aortopulmonary collaterals, or a Blalock–Taussig shunt is in place. The rare instances in which this does occur may contribute to increased mortality for Fontan-type surgery in GUCH patients.

GUCH patients with pulmonary hypertension present for anaesthesia in cardiac centres for procedures such as cardioversion, transoesophageal echocardiography and the insertion of indwelling venous lines for antibiotic therapy. In general hospital practice they may require local or general anaesthesia for a variety of procedures including appendicectomy and even caesarean section. These patients represent a very high-risk group and should be managed by experienced senior staff. The fundamental principle of management is maintaining the balance between pulmonary vascular resistance (PVR) and systemic vascular resistance (SVR). As PVR is usually fixed it is essential to avoid excessive vasodilatation and maintain right ventricular pre-load with vasoconstrictors and volume replacement. This can be monitored by central venous pressure measurements (if required). A pulmonary artery catheter may be impossible to insert in many patients with inoperable GUCH disease. It can also cause excessive dysrhythmias and provides little useful or interpretable information.

Hypoxaemia and hypercarbia should also be avoided in patients with high pulmonary pressures in case there is a reactive or reversible component of the pulmonary hypertension. For all but the shortest procedures, intubation and mechanical ventilation is desirable.

## Cyanosis

In our series of GUCH patients undergoing cardiac surgery (Dore *et al.,* 1997) those with central cyanosis had a high early mortality of 18% (9 of 49) patients. Cyanotic patients also spent a longer period in intensive care, had a longer in-hospital stay and had a significantly greater requirement for donor blood, fresh frozen plasma, cryoprecipitate and platelets. This may be because GUCH patients with cyanosis tend to have a more complex form of congenital heart disease. It also indicates, however, the profound pathological effects of cyanosis.

Patients with chronic cyanosis bleed more intra-operatively than those with a normal arterial oxygen saturation. This is due to two main problems: the presence of an extensive collateral circulation and abnormalities of haemostasis.

## Systemic to pulmonary collaterals

The presence of significant aortopulmonary collaterals should be identified angiographically prior to surgery. In some patients they are acquired and probably originate from dilated bronchial arteries. In the majority they are an integral part of the congenital abnormality, for example, as in pulmonary atresia. If the size and nature of the central pulmonary arteries are considered adequate to allow a corrective procedure, the systemic pulmonary collaterals should be embolized prior to surgery (Shore, 1994). If this is not possible they should be ligated, before establishing cardiopulmonary bypass, to prevent systemic arterial steal and persistent back-bleeding from the pulmonary artery. This may obscure the operative field and there is a danger of ventricular distension if the heart is not adequately vented. Hypothermia and low flow cardiopulmonary bypass may also be indicated in this situation.

## Haemostasis

Chronic cyanosis in GUCH patients leads to polycythaemia and abnormal haemostasis. The precise mechanism of this latter effect remains unclear but relevant factors include thrombocytopenia, platelet dysfunction, hypofibrinoge-naemia, accelerated fibrinolysis and clotting factor deficiencies. Intra-operative bleeding is further exacerbated because of a number of other factors including the presence of collaterals, heparinization and the deleterious effect of cardiopulmonary bypass on clotting mechanisms.

Meticulous surgical technique, with particular attention to haemostasis during sternotomy and chest closure, is obviously mandatory in GUCH patients with cyanotic heart disease. Donor blood and blood products should also be readily available and administered on the basis of serial estimations of the patients' haemoglobin and clotting status. Aprotinin can also be useful in minimizing intra-operative bleeding.

## Abnormal renal function

Postoperative renal impairment is particularly common in GUCH patients. Many have been chronically dependent on diuretics, have a reduced cardiac output and may have suffered renal insults during previous surgery. In our experience renal dysfunction is more common in cyanotic patients. This is not surprising, considering the deleterious effects of a high blood viscosity on renal blood flow, combined with the additional problems of hypoxia and complex surgery. Meticulous attention to fluid balance and pharmacological renal support is essential intra-operatively. Haemofiltration may be required postoperatively.

## Ventricular dysfunction

The presence of chronic pressure and volume overload in GUCH patients can lead to abnormalities of both systolic and diastolic ventricular function. Right ventricular dysfunction is often the rate-limiting step in the circulation and this needs to be assessed pre-operatively, and frequently reassessed postoperatively. In this respect echocardiography can be extremely helpful. Myocardial dysfunction is particularly common in cyanotic patients. They have a reduced ability to increase cardiac output in response to exercise and stress pre-operatively, and myocardial function can be further depressed in the immediate postoperative period. Possible mechanisms for this myocardial dysfunction include recurrent episodes of myocardial hypoxia, decreased coronary perfusion and increased blood viscosity leading to microvascular coronary occlusion. In addition, left ventricular overload occurs due to the presence of aortopulmonary collaterals, or a Blalock–Taussig shunt. Some of these patients may have also sustained a degree of myocardial damage during previous surgery and cardiopulmonary bypass.

Optimal myocardial preservation is essential during adult congenital heart surgery to minimize further deterioration of ventricular function. Effective cardioplegia regimes, combined with systemic hypothermia, remain the mainstay of myocardial protection. Prevention of ventricular distension with adequate venting techniques is also important. Residual haemodynamic defects, e.g. incomplete closure of a ventricular septal defect, a residual gradient following coarctation repair, or partially relieved pulmonary stenosis are poorly tolerated in this group of patients. Careful intra-operative assessment of the repair is therefore essential, particularly if myocardial function is poor on weaning from cardiopulmonary bypass.

## Dysrhythmias

Dysrhythmias are common in patients with GUCH disease. Atrial dysrhythmias frequently occur as a late complication of atrial surgery such as the Mustard procedure for transposition of the great arteries (TGA) and in the presence of atrial distension after a Fontan procedure. Atrial dysrhythmias can also be a late indication of conduit obstruction (usually right ventricle to pulmonary artery conduit). Postoperatively, dysrhythmias of any nature will lead to a further decrease in cardiac output. The loss of atrial transport can be particularly deleterious in this group of patients with pre-existing myocardial dysfunction.

Sequential atrioventricular pacing may be required at any stage in the post-bypass period and it is routine practice to place two atrial and two ventricular epicardial pacing wires prior to chest closure.

### Problems associated with re-operation

The major problem of a re-operation for adult congenital heart disease is re-sternotomy. Additional factors which may make the management of cardio-pulmonary bypass difficult include the presence of aortic regurgitation and large aortopulmonary collaterals. The presence of a ventricular septal defect also means there is a possibility of air reaching the arterial side of the circulation if a pulmonary artery conduit or the right ventricle is breached surgically on opening the chest.

Cardiac structures, including the aorta, right ventricle and homograft conduits, are often in close proximity to the posterior aspect of the sternum. The retrosternal space is best assessed from a CT or MRI scan. If these show that cardiac structures are adjacent to the sternum it is safer to establish cardiopulmonary bypass via the femoral vessels prior to attempting sternotomy, or at least cannulate the femoral artery and vein. Cardiopulmonary bypass is then used to support the circulation and cool the patient if vascular structures are breached. Blood lost from the sternotomy site can then be returned to the venous reservoir, via the pump suckers, as the heart is dissected out.

If there is a major risk of inadvertently entering the heart it is preferable to cool the patient on femoral–femoral bypass down to a temperature of approximately 20°C and establish circulatory arrest prior to sternotomy. Ventricular distension is a hazard of this technique if the heart fibrillates during cooling. The effects of this can be minimized by external cardiac massage, or direct venting of the left ventricle through the chest wall. If the cooling process is carried out slowly, and serum potassium levels are kept in the normal range, it is often possible to cool adults below a temperature of 25°C without ventricular fibrillation occurring.

# Principles of anaesthesia for cardiac surgery in GUCH disease

## Pre-operative preparation and premedication

It is essential to ensure hydration up to the time of surgery in patients with polycythaemia. If necessary an intravenous infusion is established the night before surgery in order to minimize the possibility of thrombotic events. Light premedication (oral temazepam) is well tolerated in this group of patients, who are usually well informed regarding their cardiac condition and proposed surgery. Heavy opioid sedation may cause unacceptable hypoxia, although this is unlikely.

We encourage close relatives of GUCH patients to accompany them to the anaesthetic room and stay during induction of anaesthesia. Surgery in the patient with GUCH disease remains high risk and this is not a time to put up psychological barriers between patient, relatives and medical staff.

## Induction of anaesthesia

Induction of anaesthesia is carried out on the lines discussed in Chapter 2, with additional consideration of specific congenital abnormalities (Baum, 1996). A slow intravenous induction, following pre-oxygenation, is quite satisfactory.

We do not usually insert central venous or arterial monitoring lines under local anaesthetic before induction. Arterial and venous access can be difficult to achieve at this point in a nervous patient and it is preferable to establish invasive monitoring once the patient is anaesthetized. This gives the anaesthetist a better chance of first-time success in placing the lines, with a low complication rate.

## Management of the airway

In the majority of cases endotracheal intubation is carried out following the administration of a non-depolarizing muscle relaxant such as pancuronium. Mechanical ventilation is then commenced in the conventional manner.

For certain procedures, such as coarctation repair, or the placement of a modified Blalock–Taussig shunt, a left-sided double lumen endobronchial tube is inserted to allow the lung on the operative side to be deflated during surgery, which is carried out via a lateral thoracotomy.

Endobronchial intubation greatly facilitates the surgery for coarctation repair and poses few problems if the patient is of a suitable size to take at least a small tube. The use of a double lumen tube during a Blalock–Taussig shunt procedure is more problematical. These patients are hypoxic from the outset and therefore may not tolerate one-lung anaesthesia. On the other hand, hypoxia may be no worse during one-lung anaesthesia than that existing pre-operatively, with the patient breathing air. The improved operating conditions can be invaluable, however, speeding up surgery and lessening damage to the retracted lung. We therefore insert double lumen endobronchial tubes in patients scheduled for shunt procedures and utilize one-lung anaesthesia when it is tolerated. There is little margin for error, however, and it may be necessary to revert to two-lung ventilation at any time.

## Vascular access and monitoring

Monitoring is established as for any major cardiac surgery. In addition external defibrillator pads are aligned across the chest wall if the operation involves re-sternotomy. This allows defibrillation of the heart if ventricular fibrillation occurs before the heart has been dissected out.

Intra-arterial pressure monitoring is usually established percutaneously with a cannula in the radial artery. It is preferable to avoid the radial artery on the side of a Blalock shunt, however, and for coarctation of the aorta a right-sided radial artery line is mandatory. If a patient has had bilateral Blalock or modified Blalock shunts (systemic arterial to pulmonary artery conduits) it may be preferable to site an arterial line in the femoral artery because the radials may not give a reliable pressure recording. The femoral artery should be avoided, however, at least on the left side, if cardiopulmonary bypass is to be instituted via the femoral vessels. Central venous lines should be inserted with extreme care in patients with GUCH disease and this procedure should not be delegated to inexperienced staff. We usually insert a quadruple lumen catheter into the internal jugular vein, with a pulmonary artery catheter sheath in the same or opposite side of the neck. This sheath is most useful for volume replacement and rapid transfusion. We rarely use pulmonary artery catheters in patients with complex GUCH disease. Internal jugular venous lines may interfere with placement of the superior vena caval bypass cannula and therefore they should not be inserted too deeply. A length of approximately 15 cm is usually satisfactory but it is important to ascertain that all the distal infusion port exits of the catheter are within the vein. Internal jugular lines may also impinge on the site of surgery if an SVC to pulmonary artery anastomosis (Glenn procedure) is planned. In this situation left internal jugular venous access may be preferable, assuming there is continuity between this vessel and the right atrium via a normally situated inominate vein. It should also be noted that there may be anatomical variants of the venous system in patients with congenital heart disease and therefore cannulation of the internal jugular vein may not be straightforward. If there is doubt about the position or patency of the internal jugular vein a hand-held ultrasound scanner can be a useful device with which to image the structure. There is little room for error in placement of central lines in patients with GUCH disease. Many of these patients have clotting deficiencies and damage to arterial structures such as the carotid and subclavian arteries in the root of the neck can be disastrous, particularly in patients requiring re-sternotomy.

## Maintenance of anaesthesia

Anaesthesia is maintained with a high-dose opioid technique combined with a volatile agent such as isoflurane. There is little merit in pursuing an early extubation policy in GUCH patients. Following prolonged surgery in this relatively young group of patients it is important to prevent awareness. For this reason we administer intravenous benzodiazepines (midazolam) and commence an infusion of propofol during the re-warming period. We also continue a propofol infusion into the postoperative period. This can also be used to minimize the possibility of hypertension which can exacerbate bleeding, particularly following a re-operation.

## Discontinuation from cardiopulmonary bypass

It is important to rewarm the patient thoroughly following a long and complex procedure. This also allows for adequate re-perfusion of the myocardium after a potentially long period of aortic cross-clamping. Ideally the heart should be re-perfused for a period of 20 min for every hour of aortic cross-clamp time. Excessive rewarming is undesirable and has been implicated in the aetiology of cerebral damage following cardiopulmonary bypass. On the other hand, a substantial temperature drop after bypass can further impair haemostatic mechanisms, exacerbate myocardial dysfunction and even cause ventricular fibrillation. This scenario is much less likely if transfused fluid is warmed, and a warm air convective heating device is in use.

Weaning from bypass often requires some degree of inotropic support initially (see Chapter 4). It is difficult to predict precisely which patient will require a significant amount of inotropic support. It is prudent, however, to have standard preparations of dopamine, adrenaline, milrinone and noradrenaline made up in advance. Transoesophageal echocardiography can be very helpful, along with the usual cardiac filling pressures, in monitoring fluid replacement and inotropic therapy.

### Postoperative management

GUCH patients, with very few exceptions, are managed in the intensive care unit postoperatively. Initial management is on the lines discussed in Chapter 5, but this is modified in relation to the specific congenital defect and type of surgery carried out. Many of these patients undergo a long period of intensive care and their complex management requires a multi-disciplinary approach. Involvement of the surgical and cardiological teams, who have extensive experience of GUCH disease, is essential.

# Aortic surgery

Although not strictly cardiac surgery, surgery involving the thoracic aorta is generally performed by cardiac surgeons. The thoracic aorta is principally affected by trauma, e.g. transection, degenerative disease such as aortic dissection, or a congenital condition such as coarctation which occasionally may not present until adult life.

### Dissection of the aorta

Aortic dissection is usually a result of cystic medial necrosis, a degenerative condition of the muscular and elastic layers of the vessel. Dissection has been classified by DeBakey into three types. In type I the dissection involves the ascending aorta, the aortic arch and the descending thoracic aorta. Type II involves the ascending aorta, and type III involves the descending aorta. Types I and II generally require emergency surgery, whereas patients with a type III dissection often may be managed conservatively in the first instance, undergoing surgery several weeks following the dissection under optimal circumstances. Aortic dissection has a very high mortality, even with appropriate medical and surgical management, and rapid assessment and careful transfer of suspected cases to a cardiothoracic unit is essential.

### Initial management

Patients with acute aortic dissection often have long-standing hypertension; this coupled with the pain and anxiety associated with acute illness may result in an exceedingly high blood pressure. As propagation of the dissection is promoted by hypertension it is mandatory to rapidly control the blood pressure. Drugs such as glyceryl trinitrate, labetalol and nitroprusside are appropriate. Labetalol is particularly useful as it also decreases the rate and force of contraction of the heart, thus reducing the effects of pulsatile flow upon propagation of the dissection.

As soon as the diagnosis is suspected (history, chest X-ray and possibly CT or MRI), invasive venous and arterial monitoring must be established and the appropriate hypotensive agents commenced. If the patient is to be transferred to another hospital, he must be accompanied by a doctor who is familiar with the drugs used and capable of adjusting the infusion rate in response to the patient's resultant heart rate and blood pressure.

Once the patient has arrived in the cardiothoracic unit the diagnosis may be confirmed with transoesophageal echocardiography preferably under general anaesthesia in theatre or the intensive care unit. Features to assess include the type of dissection and site of the intimal tear, the integrity of the aortic valve and the presence of a pericardial effusion. In types I and II, acute aortic regurgitation may be present, possibly associated with coronary disruption, myocardial ischaemia and a pericardial effusion.

### Anaesthetic management

The anaesthetist is generally involved in the primary management of patients with aortic dissection because of the need for early invasive monitoring. If an arterial line is not already *in situ*, this must be placed prior to induction of anaesthesia. Anaesthesia is then achieved with careful control of the blood pressure. If acute aortic regurgitation is suspected, afterload must be reduced and bradycardia avoided as described above. The airway is then secured. If the surgery involves the descending thoracic aorta and is to be carried via a thoracotomy, a left-sided double lumen endobronchial tube must be inserted. It should be remembered that placement of a left endobronchial tube may be difficult in the presence of a large aneurysm. If difficulty is encountered, the lower airways should be examined with a fibre-optic bronchoscope in order to exclude narrowing or ulceration associated with the aneurysm.

Additional vascular access must include at least two 14G cannulae as blood loss may be excessive, a femoral arterial line and a quadruple lumen catheter and pulmonary artery catheter within the central venous circulation.

Prior to commencement of surgery the right groin is prepared for cannulation to allow rapid institution of cardiopulmonary bypass. In types I and II dissection the femoral artery is the preferred site for cannulation as it is very easy to enter the false lumen if the ascending aorta is cannulated. It must be remembered that these patients often have a thick hypertrophic left ventricle, and ischaemia may be present secondary to coronary artery involvement, thus strict attention must be paid to the balance of myocardial oxygen supply and demand, particularly prior to bypass. Similarly effective myocardial protection is essential during cardiopulmonary bypass.

Surgery for aortic dissection is complex and may include replacement of the ascending aorta, aortic root, including the replacement of the aortic valve and reimplantation of the coronary arteries, and replacement of the arch or descending thoracic aorta. If the dissection involves the aortic arch, deep hypothermic circulatory arrest is necessary in order to perform the anastomoses of the great vessels. The replacement of the descending thoracic aorta is generally performed via a thoracotomy incision and one-lung ventilation is required.

Aortic surgery is associated with a risk of excessive peri-operative blood loss. This is due to a combination of surgical factors and the coagulopathy created by deep hypothermia. This blood loss should be anticipated by the insertion of adequate venous access, and the provision of a sufficient supply of cross-matched blood and clotting factors. The use of aprotinin is controversial if the coronary arteries are to be re-implanted.

There is a risk of paraplegia associated with surgery involving the descending thoracic aorta, due to interruption of the blood supply to the spinal cord. A significant degree of spinal cord protection may be gained by allowing the patient to cool to around 34°C. Certainly the application of surface warming to the lower limbs is absolutely contraindicated. It is also wise to provide postoperative analgesia with an intravenous opioid such as morphine, rather than insert an epidural catheter and risk the occurrence of an epidural haematoma with resulting confusion over the aetiology of any spinal cord damage.

Central to the postoperative management of these patients is the continuing control of the blood pressure, as the entire false lumen is not usually resected during surgery. Thus surges in blood pressure may predispose to continued dissection of the remaining false channel and should be avoided.

## Aortic transection

Aortic transection is a deceleration injury, usually sustained as a result of a road traffic or other high speed accident. As the aortic arch is fixed, and the heart and descending thoracic aorta are relatively mobile, the tear usually occurs either in the ascending aorta or just distal to the left subclavian artery.

It must be remembered that the chest X-ray is normal in almost 30% of patients who have an aortic transection. It is therefore important to have a high index of suspicion in patients who have suffered a deceleration injury, in order to prevent the diagnosis from being missed.

Echocardiography or aortography is generally used to confirm the presence and site of a tear. The anaesthetic management is then similar to that for aortic dissection. Emphasis is placed upon the careful control of the blood pressure, there must be sufficient venous access to allow the replacement of the often excessive blood loss, and in the case of descending thoracic aortic surgery, one-lung ventilation may be necessary to facilitate surgical access.

## Coarctation of the aorta

Coarctation of the aorta is a congenital narrowing of the descending aorta involving the site of the ductus arteriosus. This may result in severe obstruction to the aortic blood flow, poor lower body perfusion and a metabolic acidosis. Generally coarctation of the aorta is diagnosed and treated in infancy, but less severe forms may present later in childhood or in adult life. In this situation the blood flow to the lower part of the body is augmented by the development of aortic collaterals; however, upper limb hypertension and left ventricular hypertrophy are still generally present.

Surgery in adult life usually involves resection of the coarctation and an end-to-end anastomosis via a left lateral thoracotomy.

## Anaesthetic considerations

On arrival in the anaesthetic room, a right radial arterial line is sited in order to monitor upper body blood pressure during induction, surgery, and in particular during aortic cross-clamping. Following induction of anaesthesia central venous catheters and a femoral arterial line are inserted. As in the case of aortic dissection, an epidural is not sited as there is a potential risk of major blood loss in addition to cord ischaemia. During the period of aortic cross-clamping, severe upper body hypertension must be avoided as this may provoke myocardial ischaemia and a deterioration in left ventricular function. Upper body hypotension must also be avoided as the blood supply via collaterals to the lower body may be inadequate to prevent damage to the spinal cord or kidneys. As well as normotension, mild hypothermia may help to protect the spinal cord from damage during cross-clamping. Thus the patient is allowed to cool to approximately 34°C in order to maximize this protective effect.

On removal of the cross-clamp, rebound hypertension may be troublesome. Glyceryl trinitrate is a useful first line approach, but often sodium nitroprusside and intravenous beta-blockers are needed in order to bring the blood pressure under control effectively. Clearly this is vital in the early postoperative period in order to prevent bleeding from the site of anastomosis. In addition however, postoperative hypertension is also associated with bowel ischaemia due to abnormal patterns of flow in the mesenteric artery.

# Repeat cardiac surgery

The number of patients presenting for repeat cardiac surgery is increasingly progressively as the morbidity and mortality from the initial operation, be it coronary artery bypass grafting, valve replacement, congenital cardiac disease or transplantation, continues to fall. The patients undergoing repeat cardiac surgery have a higher risk of an adverse outcome, principally due to the progressive nature of cardiac disease, the need for more complex surgery, difficulties in achieving adequate myocardial protection, the increased risk of bleeding and the patient's advancing age.

## Anaesthetic management

The pre-operative anaesthetic assessment should pay particular attention to the current status of the patient and any peri-operative complications suffered by the patient around the time of his previous surgery. Sufficient blood and blood products should be requested at this stage. In our institution the premedicant of choice is temazepam administered orally 2 hours pre-operatively. If the patient is very anxious, additional midazolam may be given intravenously in the anaesthetic room. The insertion of intravenous and intra-arterial cannulae may be technically difficult, nonetheless it is essential that at least a peripheral venous line and an arterial line are inserted prior to induction.

Induction of anaesthesia should then proceed with care; particular attention should be paid to poor ventricular function, ongoing ischaemia and a slow circulation time. Following induction, the stable haemodynamic status of the patient must be maintained in accordance with their pre-existing disease as described earlier. External defibrillation paddles should be applied to the patient and blood should be checked and available in the operating theatre prior to incision, as potentially catastrophic bleeding may occur immediately following sternotomy. Drugs such as aprotinin and cell salvage techniques may also be used in these patients in order to limit what may otherwise be major peri-operative bleeding.

Patients undergoing repeat cardiac surgery also tend to have longer cross-clamp, bypass and operation times. Effective myocardial preservation is more difficult to achieve, thus the need for prolonged postoperative haemodynamic and ventilatory support is more likely. The reader is referred to Chapter 5 for further details of the postoperative care of patients undergoing cardiac surgery.

## Transplantation

Although some of the anaesthetic implications of heart and heart–lung transplantation will be discussed in this section, a detailed exposition of heart and lung transplantation is beyond the scope of this book. The author is referred to established texts for further details on this extensive subject.

### Anaesthetic management

By the nature of organization of organ harvest in this country, the anaesthetist generally meets the transplant recipient for the first time in the middle of the night. Although this is not the ideal time to perform a pre-operative visit, it is important that a thorough assessment is performed and an understanding of the severity of the patient's condition is gained. Many of these patients are undergoing repeat surgery with implications for the chest opening and the timing of the donor harvest. Also severe heart failure may result in renal and hepatic dysfunction, and the vigorous use of diuretic drugs, all of which have implications for anaesthesia. Generally, transplant patients do not receive premedication as they are often very well informed and motivated, and even a small dose of a hypnotic agent may result in a critical reduction in preload and severe hypotension.

Upon arrival in the anaesthetic room, peripheral venous and arterial access is gained. All intravascular lines and the endotracheal intubation should be performed under as aseptic conditions as possible as these patients will receive high doses of immunosuppressant drugs and will therefore be prone to infection. In the case of heart–lung transplantation a relatively large endotracheal tube is used to facilitate fibre-optic bronchoscopy postoperatively in order to inspect the suture line. In our institution we insert a quadruple lumen catheter and an 8-French sheath in the left internal jugular vein following induction of anaesthesia. This allows the preservation of the right internal jugular vein as a more direct route to the right ventricle for post-transplant endomyocardial biopsies.

Immediately following the induction of anaesthesia, cyclosporin, azathioprine and broad-spectrum antibiotics are given. The peri-operative immunosuppressant regime is currently completed by administering methylprednisolone upon removal of the aortic cross-clamp. As the ejection fraction in these patients may be little more than 15%, post-induction hypotension is common and must be treated aggressively with inotropes or vasoconstrictors. The administration of large amounts of fluid is generally inadvisable unless there are clear indications that the patient is hypovolaemic, as it will certainly precipitate worsening heart failure.

Following implantation of the donor heart, assuming adequate myocardial preservation and the avoidance of an excessive donor organ ischaemic time, separation from cardiopulmonary bypass should be achieved relatively easily. If the ischaemic time of the donor organ is greater than 4 hours there is a progressive increase in operative mortality. Whilst in transit the donor heart is protected with a potassium-based cardioplegia solution which arrests the heart in diastole. This is supplemented with topical cooling in order to maintain the myocardial temperature at 4°C. Occasionally the donor heart has pre-existing disease or has suffered a significant ischaemic insult which compromises its function and necessitates the use of inotropes or even a ventricular assist device. It is generally the right ventricle that fails in this situation due to an inability to cope with any increase in the pulmonary vascular resistance in the recipient. Transoesophageal echocardiography is a useful tool to detect the onset of right ventricular dilatation and failure. Post-bypass the heart rate is maintained at 90–100 beats/min as the denervated heart has an impaired ability to function adequately in the presence of an excessive preload. This relative tachycardia may be achieved with isoprenaline, which has the added advantage of additional beneficial pulmonary vasodilatation. An alternative useful pulmonary vasodilator in these patients is nitric oxide which may be commenced in theatre and subsequently continued in the intensive care unit. A pulmonary artery catheter may be sited via the left internal jugular vein sheath post-bypass and will provide useful information regarding the cardiac output and allow calculation of the systemic and pulmonary vascular resistance.

Excessive postoperative bleeding is a major cause of morbidity and mortality following cardiac transplantation, particularly in patients undergoing re-operation. This risk may be reduced by the use of aprotinin peri-operatively and the timely and appropriate use of blood and blood products post-bypass. Despite this the overall operative survival for heart and heart–lung transplantation is progressively improving, the current 30-day survival being in excess of 95%. This presents new challenges to the anaesthetist as more and more transplant patients are presenting for non-cardiac surgery. Also, the difficult problems of obliterative bronchiolitis, and the severe form of coronary artery disease that appears to afflict these patients are becoming more prevalent, which again have implications for the anaesthetist.

# References

Baum V.C. (1996) The adult patient with congenital disease. *J Cardiothorac Vasc Anaesth;* **10:** 261–282.

Baum V.C. and Perloff J.K. (1993) Anaesthetic implications of adult congenital heart disease. *Anesth Analg;* **76:** 1342–1358.

Dore A., Glancy L., Stone S. *et al.* (1997) Cardiac surgery for grown-up congenital heart patients: survey of 307 consecutive operations from 1991 to 1994. *Am J Cardiol;* **80:** 906–913.

Falk V., Walther T., Diegeler A. *et al.* (1996) Echocardiographic monitoring of minimally invasive mitral valve surgery using an endoaortic clamp. *J Heart Valve Dis;* **5**(6): 630–637.

Findlow D. and Doyle E. (1997) Congenital heart disease in adults. *Br J Anaesth;* **78:** 416–430.

Frazier O.H., Cooley D.A., Kadipasaoglu K.A. *et al.* (1995) Transmyocardial laser revascularization: initial clinical results. *Circulation;* **90:** S1640.

Grundeman P.F., Borst C., van Herwaarden J.A. *et al.* (1997) Haemodynamic changes during displacement of the beating heart by the Utrecht Octapus method. *Ann Thorac Surg;* **63:** S88–92.

Horvath K.A., Mannting F., Cummings N. *et al.* (1996) Transmyocardial laser revascularization: operative techniques and clinical results at two years. *J Thorac Cardiovasc Surg;* **111**(5): 1047–1052.

Hosking M.P. and Beynen F.M. (1992) The modified Fontan procedure: physiology and anaesthetic implications. *J Cardiothorac Vasc Anaesth;* **6:** 465–475.

Kaplan J.A. (1993) Thoracic aortic disease. In *Cardiac Anaesthesia*. W.B. Saunders, London, pp. 758–780.

Kirklin J.W. and Barratt-Boyes B.G. (1993) Acute aortic dissection. In *Cardiac Surgery*. Churchill Livingstone, Edinburgh, pp. 1721–1748.

Shore D.F. (1994) Surgery for congenital defects. In *Congenital Heart Disease in Adults* (Eds Reddington A., Shore D.F. and Oldershaw P.). WB Saunders, London, pp. 171–177.

Tevaearai H.T., Mueller X.M. and von Segesser L.K. (1997) Minimally invasive harvest of the saphenous vein for coronary artery bypass grafting. *Ann Thorac Surg;* **63:** S119–21.

# Chapter 4

# Cardiopulmonary bypass

## History

The astonishing advances in cardiac surgery in the latter part of this century have been possible only due to the advent of successful cardiopulmonary bypass. The first successful intracardiac operation to be carried out using a pump oxygenator was the closure of an atrial septal defect on May 6 1953. Since that time the complexity and safety of cardiopulmonary bypass has improved almost beyond recognition, allowing the performance of increasingly complex cardiovascular, respiratory and neurological procedures.

## Principles of bypass

The safety of cardiopulmonary bypass has increased greatly since the early 1950s such that for the vast majority of patients cardiac surgery has now become a low-risk procedure. The principle aim of cardiopulmonary bypass is to divert blood away from the heart, oxygenate it, remove carbon dioxide and return it to the patient to perfuse the vital organs adequately.

A typical cardiopulmonary bypass circuit consists of one or two venous cannulae inserted in the right atrium or vena cavae, a cardiotomy reservoir, a fresh gas supply with flowmeter and possibly access for an anaesthetic vaporizer, an oxygenator which may have an integral heat exchanger, a pump and an arterial cannula inserted into the ascending aorta. There are also suction devices and there may be a cardioplegia delivery system and a haemofiltration circuit. The circuit also contains several sampling ports, filters, bubble traps, and both pressure and temperature monitoring devices (Fig. 4.1).

### Cardiopulmonary bypass oxygenation systems

The blood passing through an extracorporeal circuit may be oxygenated via a bubble oxygenator or, more usually now, a membrane oxygenator. Bubble oxygenators are simple in design. Venous blood enters a mixing chamber where fresh gas passes across a screen to mix with the blood in the form of small bubbles. This is a low pressure system with a gradient of approximately 30 cm $H_2O$ and is generally sited before the pump in the bypass circuitry. The blood is subsequently defoamed by bubble filters and a silicone-based defoaming agent

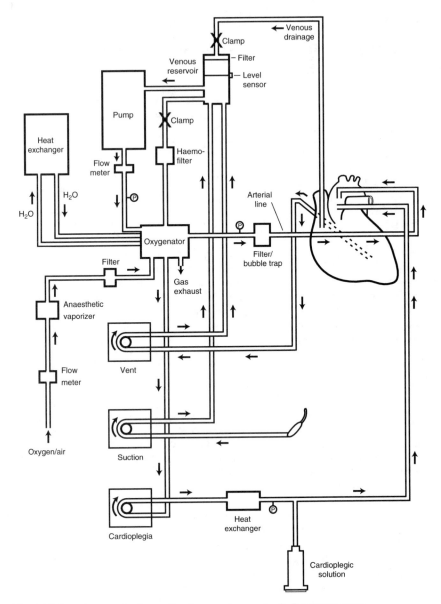

**Fig. 4.1** Schematic example of a cardiopulmonary bypass circuit. P, pressure gauge

(dimethylpolysiloxane). Bubble oxygenators also incorporate a reservoir allowing the blood to pause briefly in the circuit, so that any residual bubbles can rise to the surface.

In recent years there has been a move away from the use of bubble oxygenators towards membrane oxygenators. Indeed, a survey carried out by Silvay *et al.* in 1993 reported that 91.5% of the respondents used membrane oxygenators, compared with only 5% in 1982. The reasons for this change in practice include better gas exchange, fewer microemboli, plus a lower level of granulocyte and complement activation associated with the use of membrane oxygenators. Certainly membrane oxygenators appear to provoke less red blood cell haemolysis and to preserve platelet numbers and function better than bubble oxygenators. Also the incidence of bypass-related lung injury appears to be lower when membrane oxygenators are used.

Structurally, membrane oxygenators consist of a blood phase separated from the fresh gas flow by a membrane. This membrane may allow gas exchange only by diffusion, or it may contain micropores of less than 1 micron in diameter which allow direct mixing of the blood with the fresh gas for a short period of time following the start of bypass. The period of mixing is limited by the rapid deposition of plasma proteins on the membrane during the early phase of cardiopulmonary bypass, sealing the micropores.

The membrane used in these oxygenators is either in the form of hollow fibres or folded sheets of polypropylene. The hollow fibres may have the blood phase on the inside or the outside of the fibre; however, the latter is generally favoured as there is probably a lower risk of thrombosis within the oxygenator.

Both bubble oxygenators and membrane oxygenators usually incorporate a heat exchanger within their design to allow accurate control of the patient's temperature during surgery.

## Cardiopulmonary bypass pump systems

Cardiopulmonary bypass pumps may generate flow principally via a roller pump or a centrifugal pump, and the flow produced may be continuous or pulsatile.

### Roller pumps

In this method of extracorporeal support the blood is pushed through the tubing by a series of rollers (Fig. 4.2). These rollers may be occlusive or non-occlusive, the degree of occlusion often being adjustable. Occlusive pumps may be

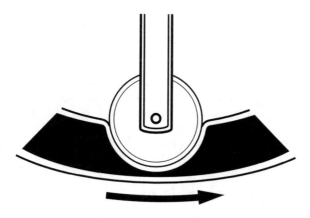

**Fig. 4.2** Cardiopulmonary bypass roller pump

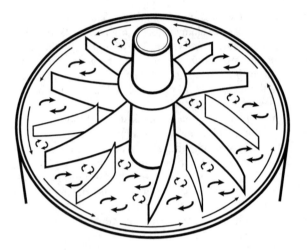

**Fig. 4.3** Cardiopulmonary bypass centrifugal pump

associated with an increased level of platelet activation and red cell damage unless carefully adjusted (Indeglia *et al.*, 1968).

### Centrifugal pumps

Centrifugal pumps create flow either by a series of rotating cones or blades (Fig. 4.3). Although expensive, this form of flow generation probably results in less platelet activation and red cell haemolysis than with roller pumps, particularly if the duration of bypass is greater than 2 hours (Parault and Conrad, 1991). Centrifugal pumps may also produce fewer gaseous and particulate microemboli (Wheeldon *et al.*, 1990; Uretzky *et al.*, 1987).

The flow generated by roller pumps may be pulsatile or non-pulsatile. In general centrifugal pumps can generate only non-pulsatile flow. It is difficult to believe that there are no benefits of improved organ function associated with physiological pulsatile flow; however, the situation remains controversial. Certainly several studies have shown that gastrointestinal perfusion is improved in the presence of pulsatile flow (Gaer *et al.*, 1994). This in turn may lead to the production of lower levels of endogenous endotoxins which have been implicated in post-bypass multiorgan failure (Watarida *et al.*, 1994). The evidence for improved cerebral perfusion with pulsatile flow, and therefore protection from hypoxia or ischaemia during cardiopulmonary bypass is, however, conflicting (Onoe *et al.*, 1994; Hindman *et al.*, 1995). It is possible that the pulsatile flow generated in the bypass circuit is not effectively transmitted to the cerebral microvasculature, resulting in difficulty in detecting any differences between the two techniques (Knothe *et al.*, 1995).

### Use of filters in cardiopulmonary bypass

Macro- and microemboli are an inherent feature of cardiopulmonary bypass. They may be particulate or gaseous and play a significant role in postoperative organ dysfunction. Thus it is important to have filters within the bypass circuitry, particularly in the arterial line, in order to trap these emboli before they reach the patient (Fig. 4.1). Filters may also be used during priming of the bypass circuitry, in the cardiotomy reservoir, between the cardiotomy reservoir and the main circuit, in the fresh gas flow line, in the blood administration sets if blood is added to the priming solution, and even in the cardioplegia delivery system.

The filters used may be divided into depth, screen and micropore filters. Depth filters consist of packed wool or foam and have no definite pore size; screen filters consist of a woven sheet with a defined pore size of between 0.2–40 microns in diameter. The micropore filters have a defined pore size of 5–40 microns. All these filters have been shown to reduce the risk of micro- and macroemboli passing to the patient, but they also contribute to the consumption of platelets during cardiopulmonary bypass. They may become blocked and may themselves become a source of microemboli. Filters can also cause haemolysis and complement activation.

## Use of vents in cardiopulmonary bypass

Venting the heart during cardiopulmonary bypass implies the decompression of one or more chambers by a cannula, or designated suction catheter. This effectively prevents distension of the ventricle and delays rewarming thus contributing to effective myocardial protection. The right heart is vented by the venous cannula if this is sited in the right atrium. The left ventricle may be vented via its apex, via the cardioplegia cannula in the aortic root (once the cardioplegia has been given), or via a catheter passed from the right superior pulmonary vein into the left atrium and across the mitral valve into the ventricle. A catheter placed in the pulmonary artery or right ventricle will also provide some degree of left ventricular venting. The vent is then attached to a roller pump and the blood aspirated is returned to the cardiotomy reservoir for reinfusion (Fig. 4.1).

## Cardiopulmonary bypass priming solutions

In the pioneering days of cardiopulmonary bypass, whole blood was used to prime the bypass circuit. It was not until the early 1960s that crystalloid solutions were introduced as a possible priming solution. Crystalloid solutions had the advantage that they resulted in significant haemodilution at the commencement of bypass thus reducing the viscosity of the circulating fluid so that organ perfusion was maintained even in the presence of profound hypothermia. This improvement in perfusion resulted in a decrease in post-bypass complications including renal, pulmonary and neurological dysfunction.

Currently, 1.5–2.0 L of a crystalloid solution such as Ringer's lactate is commonly used to prime an adult bypass circuit. To this 5000 units of heparin is generally added (Hett et al., 1994). A colloid solution such as albumin or hetastarch may also be added to raise the oncotic pressure of the prime and limit postoperative oedema. The use of glucose-containing fluids is controversial as, although glucose may reduce peri-operative fluid requirements, hyperglycaemia has been implicated in worsening ischaemia-related cerebral damage (Metz, 1995; Hindman, 1995).

Certain drugs may be added to the prime in specific circumstances, including calcium chloride, mannitol, aprotinin and corticosteroids. Oxygen-carrying solutions such as perflurocarbons and haemoglobin solutions are currently under evaluation as useful additions to the priming solution. It is hoped that by increasing the oxygen-carrying capacity of the prime it will be possible to tolerate lower haematocrits and reduce the need for peri-operative blood transfusion.

In the majority of patients the inevitable haemodilution associated with cardiopulmonary bypass is corrected by a vigorous diuresis that occurs in the early postoperative period. However, in the presence of extreme haemodilution, a large circulating volume or poor renal function, haemofiltration during cardio-pulmonary bypass may be necessary to avoid postoperative anaemia, oedema and increased organ dysfunction. The haemofilter consists of a semipermeable membrane which allows filtration of molecules up to 20 000 daltons. Thus small molecules such as sodium and potassium are freely filtered, as are heparin and some other drugs which therefore may require supplementation. Clotting factors and the formed elements of blood are not filtered, thus as well as increasing the haematocrit, haemofiltration helps to preserve the integrity of the coagulation system.

The haemofilter is integrated into the bypass circuit via a shunt distal to the pump which provides the driving force across the membrane. The filtrate is discarded and the haemoconcentrated blood returned to the cardiotomy reservoir.

## Pre-bypass period

The maintenance of adequate coronary perfusion with appropriate preload and afterload management is vital in the immediate pre-bypass period. This is often a time when there may be considerable haemodynamic instability, particularly during the surgical cannulation of the great vessels, and constant vigilance on the part of the anaesthetist is essential. The reader is referred to Chapter 3 for further details of the management of patients with specific conditions during the pre-bypass period.

## Heparinization regimes

Contact between blood and the artificial surface of the bypass circuit results in massive activation of the clotting and complement cascades, therefore an anticoagulant, most commonly heparin, is given in order to prevent potentially fatal coagulation at the commencement of bypass. Heparin is a highly sulphated polyanionic (negatively charged) mucopolysaccharide with a molecular weight between 3000 and 40 000 daltons (mean approximately 15 000 daltons). It acts principally by potentiating the activity of antithrombin III. Antithrombin III in turn inhibits the activity of thrombin and factors IXa, Xa, XIa and XIIa, thus inhibiting clot formation (Fig. 4.4).

Traditionally heparin is given in a dose of 300 IU/kg via a central vein immediately prior to cannulation of the great vessels. The activated clotting time measured from a radial arterial sample reaches a plateau within 1 min (Gravlee *et al.,* 1988), thus allowing rapid confirmation of the presence of heparin in the system prior to commencing cardiopulmonary bypass.

INTRINSIC PATHWAY                    EXTRINSIC PATHWAY

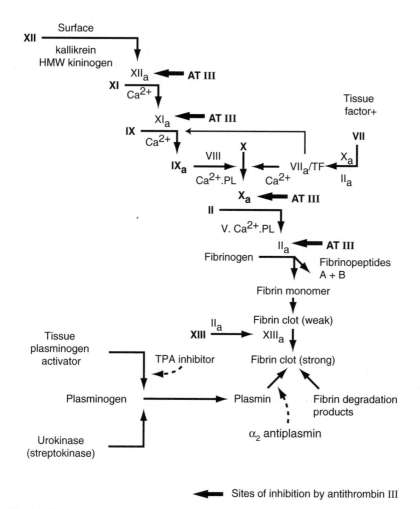

**Fig. 4.4** Clotting cascade with particular reference to sites inhibited by antithrombin III (AT III)

The heparin should not be given by peripheral intravenous injection, as during surgery it is difficult to confirm reliably that the cannula is correctly positioned within a vein; also, in the presence of a low cardiac output the onset of action may be delayed. The elimination half-life of heparin is variable, being dependent upon many factors including the dose given, the temperature and renal function of the patient. Thus regular assessments of heparin activity are carried out during the bypass period, usually by means of the activated clotting time, although more accurate heparin assay systems are now becoming available. An activated clotting time of greater than 480 sec, or three times the baseline value is considered adequate to prevent coagulation during cardiopulmonary bypass.

Recently, however, the dose of heparin given during cardiac surgery has been increasingly called into question. A standard dose of 300 IU/kg produces widely varying, and often inadequate, plasma levels of heparin in different patients. Also the activated clotting time bears no relationship to the actual plasma heparin level during bypass and is therefore a very poor measure of the adequacy of anticoagulation. The advent of heparin-bonded bypass circuitry has further complicated the issue, as it is not clear what plasma levels of heparin are necessary in this situation. Certainly there appears to be significantly less cellular activation and thrombin generation during bypass when heparin-bonded circuitry is used (Bannan et al., 1997). It is likely, however, that the principle site for clotting factor activation is within the pericardium which is not affected by heparin bonding of the bypass circuit (Chung et al., 1996; Philippou et al., 1997).

As well as the activation of the clotting system during cardiopulmonary bypass, contact between the circulating blood and the non-physiological surface of the bypass circuitry results in activation of the complement cascade, principally via the alternative pathway. This results in cell lysis, vasodilatation, histamine release, chemotaxis of neutrophils and macrophages and increased capillary permeability. It is this inflammatory reaction that is responsible for much of the organ damage that occurs post cardiopulmonary bypass.

## Management of cardiopulmonary bypass

Cardiopulmonary bypass is commenced by blood being drained from the patient via one or more venous cannulae in the right atrium or vena cavae; the pump is commenced and the blood and priming solution is simultaneously returned to the patient via the arterial cannula sited in the ascending aorta. The flow required to maintain homeostasis during bypass is principally dependent upon the oxygen consumption of the patient. This in turn is related to age, body surface area and temperature and is approximately 4 ml/kg/min in the adult. Although there is no universally accepted value for the flow rate required during bypass to maintain normal organ perfusion, there is experimental and clinical evidence that 2.2–2.5 L/min/m$^2$ is adequate in normothermic adults (Kirklin and Barratt-Boyes, 1986). A reduction in arterial pH or central venous oxygen saturation may indicate to the perfusionist that the calculated flow is inadequate for that patient and prompt him to increase it.

Similarly, there is no universally accepted value for the optimum perfusion pressure during bypass. Historically the mean perfusion pressure has generally been maintained at between 50 and 70 mmHg. A minimum of 50 mmHg was established because is was easily attainable. By reducing collateral blood flow it provided good operating conditions, minimized the damage to blood elements caused by the bypass circuitry, and also represented the lower limit of cerebral blood flow autoregulation (Hartman, 1997). Indeed, it has been shown that if the perfusion pressure falls much below 50–55 mmHg there is an associated fall in cerebral haemoglobin oxygenation (Tamura and Tamura, 1994). It should be remembered that patients undergoing cardiac surgery are characteristically older and sicker that the normal population and may have co-existent hypertension or cerebrovascular disease, necessitating a higher perfusion pressure. Gold et al. (1995) demonstrated a decreased combined neurological and cardiac morbidity in patients managed with a mean arterial pressure of 80–100 mmHg during cardiopulmonary bypass, compared with those managed with a mean arterial pressure of 50–60 mmHg.

Manipulation of the perfusion pressure to a desired level may be achieved with vasoconstrictor and vasodilator drugs. Phenylephrine, methoxamine and metaraminol are commonly used to increase the perfusion pressure via their alpha receptor agonist effects. If the perfusion pressure is considered too high, it is essential to confirm an adequate depth of anaesthesia and analgesia before using a vasodilator agent, e.g. glyceryl trinitrate or phentolamine, to reduce the pressure.

As bypass is generally commenced in adults with an asanguinous prime there is an immediate fall in systemic vascular resistance. This is due to the reduction in viscosity of the circulating blood as a direct result of haemodilution. According to the Hagen–Poiseuille equation (Flow = $pi(P_1 - P_2)r^4/8L$ viscosity) results in a fall in the mean arterial pressure. Fortunately this effect is generally transient and the reduction in perfusion pressure is usually short lived. The perfusion pressure then gradually increases as bypass continues, due to a progressive rise in systemic vascular resistance secondary to the steady extravascular absorption of the circulating fluid.

The other pressures monitored during cardiopulmonary bypass including central venous pressure, left atrial pressure and pulmonary artery pressure, should be maintained close to zero. In particular central venous pressure may be slightly negative; any rise may indicate impaired venous drainage due to kinking or obstruction of the venous line, a malpositioned venous cannula or one of inadequate size, or an insufficient pressure drop between the patient and the venous reservoir. The resultant rise in central venous pressure will compromise the perfusion of vital organs, in particular the brain, liver and kidneys (Gravlee et al., 1993) and increase postoperative oedema as fluid is driven into the extravascular compartment. It is thus vitally important that a raised central venous pressure should not be assumed to be artefactual until all possibility of impaired venous drainage has been excluded.

## Temperature management during cardiopulmonary bypass

Hypothermia is used during cardiopulmonary bypass in order to reduce the oxygen requirements of the tissues, at a time when the perfusion of vital organs may be compromised. Blood and surface cooling are used to achieve the necessary reduction in core temperature (33–35°C mild hypothermia, 28–32°C moderate hypothermia and 22–27°C profound hypothermia). The associated decrease in tissue oxygen consumption may then allow utilization of lower flow rates if necessary. The use of lower flow rates has several potential benefits. It may facilitate surgery, decrease the blood cellular damage due to the mechanical effects of the pump–oxygenator system, decrease the rate of myocardial rewarming via non-coronary collaterals thus improving the quality of the myocardial protection, and reduce the embolic load to vital organs such as the brain.

It is now generally accepted that between 2 and 5°C of central nervous system cooling confers a significant neuroprotective effect in terms of reducing cerebral oxygen consumption and facilitating the use of lower flows. It therefore seems strange that there appears to be little difference in the incidence of cer-

**Table 4.1 Disadvantages of hypothermia during cardiopulmonary bypass**

Hypothermia impairs coagulation and promotes heparin rebound

Sludging of red blood cells may occur if the degree of haemodilution is not adequate resulting in impaired microcirculation

Hypothermia complicates the interpretation of blood gas analysis

Hypothermia impairs glucose metabolism with a tendency to hyperglycaemia

Hypothermia promotes electrolyte imbalance – myocardial cells tend to lose potassium and gain sodium at temperatures less than 32°C

Rewarming may be prolonged; hypothermia prolongs the duration of bypass and predisposes to acidosis and postoperative shivering

Rewarming may be uneven leading to regional ischaemia

Drug metabolism is altered

Cold agglutinins may be present which will cause haemolysis during hypothermia

Hypothermia predisposes to arrhythmias

Glomerular filtration is reduced, sodium, water and glucose resorption are impaired, hydrogen ion excretion is reduced and polyuria occurs, leading to potential problems with fluid balance

Hypothermia causes gastric dilatation, ileus and submucosal gastric erosions and haemorrhages

Circulating free fatty acids are increased which may further predispose to arrhythmias

---

ebrovascular damage in patients who undergo cardiopulmonary bypass at normothermia or hypothermia (Christakis *et al.*, 1995). This perhaps may be explained by the fact that the three main mechanisms of cerebral ischaemic injury during bypass are known to be macro- and microemboli, hypoperfusion and the inflammatory response described above. Embolic phenomena form by far the most important of these three categories. Emboli occur principally during aortic cross-clamping, at the start of bypass, on removal of the cross-clamp, positioning of the side-biting clamp and on removal of the aortic cannula at the end of bypass. All these events occur at normothermia, not at a time when hypothermia is present and able to confer additional cerebral protection.

Despite the obvious benefits of hypothermia, there are also significant disadvantages (Table 4.1). This has prompted the development of techniques involving normothermic cardiopulmonary bypass, which has been achieved without an apparent increase in morbidity or mortality (Tonz *et al.*, 1993).

## Acid–base management during cardiopulmonary bypass

According to Dalton's law, the solubility of a gas in a liquid is dependent upon the temperature. Thus in the case of blood, as the temperature is reduced, carbon dioxide becomes more soluble therefore its partial pressure decreases and the pH of the blood rises. During hypothermic cardiopulmonary bypass, two alternative blood–gas management strategies may be used, namely pH-stat or alpha-stat.

pH-stat management requires the addition of carbon dioxide to the blood as the partial pressure of carbon dioxide in the blood decreases with decreasing temperature. The carbon dioxide is added to the oxygenator gas flows so that when the blood gas is corrected for temperature the pH remains in the range of 7.35–7.45 and the total stores of carbon dioxide are increased.

During alpha-stat management, the total stores of carbon dioxide are maintained at a constant level, no further carbon dioxide is added to the blood and the pH, corrected for temperature, is allowed to increase as the temperature decreases. If the blood gas is measured without correction for hypothermia, its pH is also maintained in the 7.35–7.45 range. Thus, blood managed with an alpha-stat regimen is relatively alkalotic when compared with that managed with a pH-stat regimen. The relative difference between the two is dependent upon the degree of hypothermia. The term alpha refers to the uncharged fraction of the imidazole group of histidine which provides the majority of the intracellular buffering capacity. This remains constant during alpha-stat management, i.e. the proportion of positive to negative charges within the cell does not change.

In the early days of cardiopulmonary bypass pH-stat management was principally used as it was thought to help maintain cerebral blood flow by inducing cerebral vasodilatation. Although this increased cerebral blood flow has the potential disadvantage of increasing the risk of macro- and microemboli to the brain, the vasodilatation does allow improved cerebral cooling, and therefore potentially superior cerebral protection.

Conversely, although conclusive evidence is still lacking, the maintenance of intracellular neutrality is known to be essential for the normal functioning of enzymes and ultimately the integrity of the cell membrane. Thus alpha-stat management, which maintains a constant intracellular buffering capacity may be preferable. Indeed poiklothermic animals who are subject to wide ranges of body temperature follow an alpha-stat management system.

Thus it is probable that under most circumstances alpha-stat management is preferable. Prior to a period of circulatory arrest, however, the quality of cerebral cooling, and therefore the reduction in cerebral oxygen consumption becomes of paramount importance, in which case the vasodilatory action of pH-stat management is desirable. As this strategy allows the development of an intracellular acidosis, the period of pH-stat cooling is often followed by a period of alpha-stat management to help eliminate acidosis and improve cerebral metabolic recovery.

In reality, during moderate hypothermia, there is probably little difference between these two strategies in terms of morbidity and mortality following cardiopulmonary bypass. Numerous outcome studies have failed to show one technique superior to the other (Bashein *et al.*, 1990), and further research is necessary to shed more light upon this complex and controversial area.

## Management of serum electrolytes during cardiopulmonary bypass

The maintenance of serum electrolytes within the normal range during cardiopulmonary bypass is essential. This is particularly important in the case of potassium. Factors predisposing to hypokalaemia during cardiopulmonary bypass include the pre-bypass potassium concentration, hypothermia, the nature of the priming and cardioplegic solutions, and polyuria. Perhaps not surprisingly hypokalaemia is more common and severe in patients undergoing valvular surgery than those undergoing coronary artery bypass grafts, as these patients are more likely to have received intensive pre-operative diuretic therapy. If possible hypokalaemia should be corrected during bypass in order to achieve a serum potassium concentration of 4.5–5.0 mmol/L. Hyperkalaemia is less common but may occur if renal function is impaired or multiple doses of potassium-containing cardioplegia are used.

There is also a decrease in the ionized serum calcium and magnesium levels during cardiopulmonary bypass as a result of haemodilution. In the case of calcium, although calcium salts are often given at the termination of bypass, in adults this practice is not only unnecessary, it may also be deleterious, as calcium has been implicated in reperfusion injury. Conversely in the case of magnesium, the fall in serum levels during bypass may be clinically significant, predisposing towards post-bypass cardiac arrhythmias. Thus the administration of magnesium sulphate 1–2 g prior to terminating bypass may be beneficial.

It is widely accepted that hyperglycaemia exacerbates ischaemic brain injury. Thus the management of serum glucose is also important during cardiopulmonary bypass, particularly in the presence of normothermic bypass, cerebral hypoperfusion, or if circulatory arrest is employed (Hindman, 1995). Therefore glucose-containing fluids are not given prior to bypass unless hypoglycaemia is present, and the serum glucose concentration is maintained at less than 10 mmol/L for the duration of cardiopulmonary bypass. The administration of post-bypass glucose may, however, play a role in limiting reperfusion injury by helping to maintain stores of high energy phosphates at a critical time. Thus it is then advantageous to provide a constant supply of glucose at this stage by diluting any vasoactive drugs infused in a glucose-containing solution, and by using dextrose saline as the postoperative maintenance fluid.

## Anaesthesia during cardiopulmonary bypass

Adequate anaesthesia must be maintained during cardiopulmonary bypass to prevent awareness. In order to achieve this consistently, a knowledge of the effects of bypass on the pharmacokinetics of the drugs used is essential. For example, as bypass is commenced haemodilution occurs, and the pharmacokinetics of the drugs used changes, principally by a reduction in the plasma concentration. Conversely, alterations in renal and hepatic perfusion may reduce the clearance of certain drugs and cause the plasma concentration to rise steadily, and furthermore some drugs are actually absorbed by the bypass circuitry.

Anaesthesia may be maintained with a volatile agent such as isoflurane. The vaporizer is easily incorporated into the fresh gas flow of the bypass circuit and the expired vapour concentration may be monitored with a gas analyser attached to the waste gas port of the oxygenator. Several studies have shown that blood isoflurane levels achieved by this method are somewhat lower than those reached when the isoflurane is delivered via the lungs. This is possibly due to differences in uptake of isoflurane from the bypass circuit, compared with the uptake from the lungs (Loomis et al., 1986). The significance of this effect may be limited by the reduced isoflurane requirement associated with hypothermia if this is employed during bypass.

Alternatively an intravenous agent such as propofol may be used to maintain anaesthesia during cardiopulmonary bypass. This must be delivered via a central vein to ensure the reliability of administration. The concentration of propofol has been show to decrease exponentially with the duration of bypass due to sequestration by the cardiopulmonary bypass circuit (Su *et al.*, 1996), although clinically this does not generally result in increased requirements.

It may also be necessary to supplement anaesthesia with additional increments of opioids and neuromuscular blocking agents during cardiopulmonary bypass. In particular, fentanyl is sequestered in the lungs and by the oxygenator membrane, so the plasma levels may decrease dramatically at the commencement of bypass. Subsequently the half-life of fentanyl may be prolonged due to a reduction in hepatic perfusion both during and post-bypass (Koska *et al.*, 1981). A newer potent opioid, remifentanil, also shows a significant reduction in metabolism during hypothermic cardiopulmonary bypass, but because its half-life is so short accumulation does not occur and its duration of action remains entirely predictable.

## Cerebral function monitoring during cardiopulmonary bypass

Attempts to monitor cerebral function during cardiopulmonary bypass have been made since it first became apparent that bypass could be associated with postoperative neurological dysfunction. Traditionally the electroencephalogram (EEG) was used, but this fell out of favour as different anaesthetic agents were discovered to produce different effects; also, considerable expertise was required to interpret the results. Cerebral function monitors (CFAM) were then developed in which blocks of EEG data were subjected to Fourier analysis to provide trends in the fundamental frequencies. From these trends, information could be gained during bypass about cerebral hypoxia and the depth of anaesthesia. This equipment, however, remained cumbersome and its use gradually declined. More recently the measurement of jugular venous oxygen saturation, transcranial Doppler and near infra-red spectroscopy have all been used to provide useful information about cerebral function during cardiopulmonary bypass.

## Myocardial preservation

During cardiopulmonary bypass a cross-clamp is applied to the aorta and the heart rendered ischaemic. This allows good visualization of the surgical field, and facilitates a good technical result. Without adequate myocardial protection, this period of ischaemia can lead to extensive cardiac damage and a low cardiac output state postoperatively. If the patient survives, the duration of hospital stay is likely to be prolonged and long-term recovery may be complicated by late onset myocardial fibrosis.

Myocardial protection is therefore of paramount importance to the success of the procedure. There are many techniques available, each with inherent advantages and disadvantages, some of which will be mentioned here. An extensive discussion is, however, beyond the scope of this book and the reader is referred to well-established texts on this subject.

### Crystalloid versus blood cardioplegia

Crystalloid cardioplegic arrest utilizing potassium-containing solutions (Table 4.2) revolutionized myocardial protection. Hyperkalaemic cardioplegia causes myocardial membrane depolarization and diastolic cardiac arrest thus reducing the myocardial oxygen demand to a minimum, and affording considerable

**Table 4.2 Composition of a typical crystalloid cardioplegia solution**

| | |
|---|---|
| Sodium | 147 |
| Potassium | 20 |
| Magnesium | 16 |
| Calcium | 2 |
| Procaine | 1 |
| Chloride | 204 |

Values are in mmol/L

protection against the effects of ischaemia. Crystalloid cardioplegia does not however prevent abnormal transmembrane ion fluxes with the influx of calcium and chloride and the continued activity of energy-requiring calcium and sodium pumps. These contribute to the depletion of vital energy supplies and the development of intracellular calcium overload, which is thought to be critical in the development of myocardial stunning (Cohen *et al.,* 1995). Other techniques and solutions have been investigated with blood cardioplegia emerging as the most commonly used protective strategy in the United States. The advantages of blood cardioplegia include the capacity to deliver oxygen, buffering capacity and antioxidants to the myocardium at this critical time (Buckberg, 1995).

### Cold versus warm cardioplegia

Many of the problems associated with potassium-containing crystalloid cardio-plegia may be resolved by simultaneously utilizing the protective effects of myocardial cooling. Hypothermia reduces myocardial oxygen demand and therefore delays the development of ischaemic damage. The areas of the heart most at risk from increased oxygen demand as the heart rewarms are the outer half of the left ventricle, the right ventricle and the atria. Topical cooling of the heart has therefore been shown to improve myocardial protection, especially in the presence of coronary artery disease, although the application of topical iced saline is also associated with postoperative phrenic nerve palsy.

Of course, the benefits of myocardial hypothermia may also be used in conjunction with blood cardioplegia, but the increasing viscosity of the blood may limit these as it cools. Warm blood cardioplegia has also been used, and is thought to reduce reperfusion injury by limiting calcium flux into the cells, buffering the acidosis and replenishing ATP stores. Despite this, warm blood cardioplegia has not gained wide acceptance as it necessarily precludes the well-recognized neuro- and cardioprotective effects of hypothermia.

### Multidose versus single dose

Anatomically, all hearts have a significant non-coronary collateral blood flow; this allows the progressive warming of the heart and replacement of the protective cardioplegic solution with systemic blood. This fact promoted the introduction of multidose cardioplegia and the topical application of iced solutions to the heart. In a multidose technique half the original dose of cardioplegia is typically administered every 30 min of ischaemic time to replenish the cardioplegia as it is diluted by the non-coronary blood flow.

### Antegrade versus retrograde perfusion

The degree of protection conferred by any cardioplegic solution is dependent upon it reaching all the areas of the myocardium in sufficient dose to have an effect. Anterograde delivery may be via a cannula in the ascending aorta or directly into the coronary ostia. Effective delivery of cardioplegia via the ascending aorta is dependent upon the presence of a competent aortic valve, and the generation of an aortic root pressure of at least 60 mmHg in order to provide sufficient coronary flow. In the presence of coronary artery disease, particularly if important vessels are completely occluded, it may not be possible to provide sufficient coronary flow with anterograde perfusion alone. Additional retrograde coronary perfusion via the coronary sinus may therefore provide more uniform myocardial protection. To avoid potential damage, the pressure generated in the coronary sinus should not be more than 30–40 mmHg.

### Cross-clamp fibrillation

Intermittent aortic cross-clamping and induced ventricular fibrillation may be used as an alternative to cardioplegia-based myocardial protection techniques for coronary artery bypass surgery. It is thought that brief periods of ischaemia followed by reperfusion may reduce the risk of subsequent myocardial infarction. It has certainly been shown that such ischaemic preconditioning reduces the release of troponin T, a useful biochemical marker of myocardial damage (Alkhulaifi, 1997). During surgery, the preconditioning occurs whilst the cross-clamp is applied to the aorta, ventricular fibrillation is induced, and the distal anastomosis performed. The heart is then defibrillated and reperfusion is allowed to occur during the completion of proximal anastomosis. Preconditioning allows the preservation of myocardial ATP and may be associated with improved postoperative ventricular function. However, in the presence of a severely diseased ascending aorta, multiple applications of the cross-clamp may increase the risk of atheromatous emboli being released into the circulation. Direct inspection by the surgeon, and transoesophageal echocardiography of the ascending aorta, can be used to exclude the presence of a significant atheromatous plaque in the ascending aorta, which would contraindicate this technique.

## Weaning from cardiopulmonary bypass

As surgery nears completion, the patient is rewarmed to a nasopharyngeal or oesophageal temperature of 37°C. If a peripheral temperature probe is also in use the core–peripheral gap should be less than 7°C and the patient's skin should feel warm to touch. If rewarming prior to weaning from cardiopulmonary bypass is inadequate, significant further heat loss may occur while the chest is being closed. This in turn may lead to shivering, increased peripheral resistance and increased oxygen consumption, all highly undesirable in the early postoperative period. Ventricular fibrillation may occur during rewarming. This requires

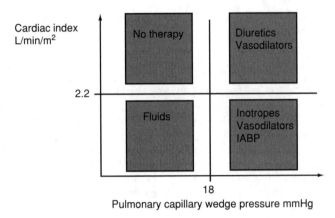

**Fig. 4.5** Schematic representation of the management of the failing heart

cardioversion with 10–30 Joules DC shock applied to the ventricles via internal defibrillator paddles. If atrial fibrillation occurs, 5–10 Joules may be similarly applied to the atria.

Rewarming to a nasopharyngeal temperature greater than 38°C is potentially as deleterious as persistent hypothermia. Grocott *et al.* in 1997 showed that the nasopharyngeal temperature upon rewarming consistently underestimates the jugular venous temperature by as much as 3.4°C. Thus the brain may be exposed to periods of significant hyperthermia, possibly increasing the risk of neurological injury associated with cardiopulmonary bypass.

If an intracardiac procedure has been performed, e.g. valve replacement, one or more of the chambers of the heart are opened to the atmosphere. In order to reduce the risk of air embolus it is important to evacuate any air from the heart before it is allowed to eject. Although air may accumulate anywhere within the heart, common sites include the left atrial appendage, along the interatrial septum and in the pulmonary veins. De-airing techniques comprise ventilation of the lungs while blood and air is aspirated via a needle and syringe from the left ventricle, aortic root, pulmonary veins and the left atrial appendage. A vent may be placed at the highest point in the ascending aorta and the heart manipulated in order to allow any air to escape. The patient may also be placed in the Trendelenburg position prior to the removal of the cross-clamp so that any air remaining is encouraged to pass up the descending aorta rather than down into the cerebral circulation. Transoesophageal echocardiography is useful in assisting de-airing as air within the heart is highly echogenic and easily detected.

The placement of temporary epicardial pacing wires may be necessary following bypass to protect against deleterious arrhythmias related to pre-existing conduction defects, drugs, incomplete myocardial protection or surgical damage to the conducting system. Ventricular, atrial or sequential pacing may be used. Ventricular pacing is indicated in the presence of long-standing atrial fibrillation or if atrial activity is absent. Atrial pacing may be used in the presence of a bradycardia if atrioventricular conduction is intact, and sequential pacing is used if atrioventricular block is present.

Finally, prior to the weaning of cardiopulmonary bypass it is vital to correct any acid–base or electrolyte imbalance present, in particular hypo- or hyperkalaemia. Ventilation is recommenced and anaesthesia, analgesia and neuromuscular blockade must be reassessed and supplemented as necessary. All monitors should be functioning correctly and any necessary myocardial support instituted.

## Separation from cardiopulmonary bypass

Once all these factors have been addressed and the patient is warm with a stable cardiac rhythm, weaning from cardiopulmonary bypass may be commenced. Initially the venous line is partially clamped and the heart is allowed to fill. Then the pump speed is reduced, allowing the heart to eject. If the blood pressure is maintained at this stage, then the venous line is fully clamped. When the heart appears to be appropriately filled and functioning well, the pump is stopped and weaning from cardiopulmonary bypass is complete. Subsequent filling of the heart may be continued via the arterial line as necessary.

The rate of weaning from bypass is dependent upon the adequacy of ventricular function. If ventricular function is poor, the period of partial bypass may be prolonged, whilst the degree of filling, heart rate and the use of inotropes are optimized. It is important at this stage to avoid distension of the heart as this results in detrimental subendocardial ischaemia. Myocardial distension may best be avoided by the direct observation of the heart by the anaesthetist and surgeon. Good communication between all members of the team at this time is crucial.

## The failing heart

Occasionally, despite careful preparation, weaning from cardiopulmonary bypass is unsuccessful, and without support the patient is unable to maintain an adequate cardiac output. The causes for this include poor pre-operative ventricular function, inadequate myocardial protection, a prolonged cross-clamp time, or an imperfect surgical repair. Other factors such as electrolyte imbalance, acidosis and arrhythmias may be implicated here and should have already been corrected.

As soon as it becomes apparent that the patient is unable to maintain an adequate cardiac output following bypass, the aetiology must be rapidly sought and appropriate therapy instituted. In less severe cases of cardiac failure, the aetiology may be obvious following a simple clinical assessment. For example, merely by observing the heart it is possible to make a crude assessment of ventricular function. Similarly, evidence of hypovolaemia or excessive vasodilatation may be gained from the surgeon by palpating the pulmonary artery wall tension.

In patients with severe post-bypass cardiac failure, a more objective assessment of haemodynamic status is necessary in order to guide treatment effectively. If not already *in situ,* a pulmonary artery flotation catheter should be inserted, and assessment of the cardiac output and pulmonary capillary wedge pressure (PCWP) made. This allows the rapid calculation of a variety of physiological variables including the cardiac index, stroke volume, and systemic and pulmonary vascular resistance. If the cardiac index and the PCWP are known, a simple scheme such as that shown in Fig. 4.5 may be used to optimize cardiac function. It may be necessary to re-institute partial or full bypass whilst fluids, inotropes and other vasoactive infusions are commenced.

## Inotropic support

Inotropic drugs improve ventricular performance at the expense of increasing myocardial oxygen consumption. As many inotropic drugs also alter the systemic and pulmonary vascular resistance they are often used in conjunction with vasoactive agents such as glyceryl trinitrate or noradrenaline in order to optimize the circulation. The inotropic and vasoactive drugs commonly used post-cardiopulmonary bypass are shown in Table 4.3; further details of their use may be found in Chapter 5.

**Table 4.3 Inotropic and vasoactive drugs commonly used post cardiopulmonary bypass**

| Drug | Indication | Effects | Dose (mcg/kg/min) |
|------|-----------|---------|-------------------|
| Adrenaline | Moderate to severe ventricular failure | Increased contractility, heart rate and systemic vascular resistance | 0.01–0.6 |
| Noradrenaline | Excessive systemic vasodilatation | Increased systemic vascular resistance | 0.01–0.3 |
| Dopamine | Mild to moderate ventricular failure, poor renal perfusion | Increased contractility, heart rate, splanchnic perfusion and systemic vascular resistance | 3–10 |
| Dobutamine | Mild to moderate ventricular failure | Increased contractility and heart rate, decreased systemic vascular resistance | 5–20 |
| Dopexamine | Moderate ventricular failure, poor renal perfusion | Increased contractility and heart rate, decreased systemic vascular resistance | 0.5–6.0 |
| Enoximone | Moderate to severe ventricular failure | Increased contractility, decreased systemic and pulmonary vascular resistance | 5–20 |
| Milrinone | Moderate to severe ventricular failure | Increased contractility, decreased systemic and pulmonary vascular resistance | 0.35–0.75 |
| Glyceryl trinitrate | Excessive pulmonary and systemic vasoconstriction, poor coronary perfusion | Increased coronary perfusion and venodilatation | 0.1–10 |
| Sodium nitroprusside | Excessive pulmonary and systemic vasoconstriction | Decreased systemic vascular resistance | 0.5–10 |
| Isoprenaline | Bradycardia and heart block | Increased heart rate, decreased systemic vascular resistance | 0.01–0.1 |

## Mechanical support for the failing heart

Occasionally even with optimal filling and appropriate inotropic therapy, ventricular function is insufficient to maintain an adequate circulation. In this situation various devices are available to provide mechanical support for the failing heart. These can offer a range of support, from decreasing the work performed by the ventricle to functionally replacing it.

Following cardiopulmonary bypass if it becomes apparent that the cardiac output is inadequate, the first step is to reinstitute bypass in order to allow a period of cardiac reperfusion and the optimization of inotropic therapy prior to considering more complex devices. It must be remembered that these devices, in general, only offer a short-term solution, allowing time for the ventricle to recover or providing a bridge to transplantation.

## Intra-aortic balloon counterpulsation

The intra-aortic balloon pump (IABP) was introduced in 1962, and remains a popular method for treating cardiogenic shock, including that which occurs post-cardiopulmonary bypass. The device consists of a balloon tipped catheter inserted via the femoral artery into the aorta, so that the tip is positioned just distal to the origin of the left subclavian artery (Fig. 4.6). The radial or brachial pulse should always be palpated in the left arm following placement to ensure that the tip of the balloon has not entered or occluded the subclavian artery. Transoesophageal echocardiography is also useful in confirming the correct placement of the tip.

The inflation of the balloon should be timed to occur at the dicrotic notch of the arterial pressure wave; this in turn corresponds with the peak of the T wave

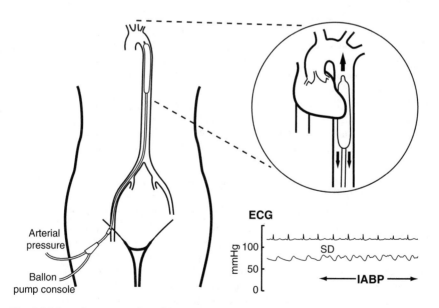

**Fig. 4.6** Schematic representation of intra-aortic balloon counterpulsation

on the ECG (Fig. 4.6). Thus inflation takes place during diastole and deflation during systole, providing a wave of counterpulsation in the aorta. This counterpulsation increases the mean diastolic aortic pressure, which in turn improves organ blood flow, in particular coronary and cerebral perfusion. There is also a modest reduction in systolic arterial pressure reducing the left ventricular afterload (Nanas and Moulopoulos, 1994). The counterpulsation thus results in improvements in the myocardial oxygen supply, endocardial viability and cardiac output.

If inflation of the balloon occurs before the dicrotic notch, afterload is increased, whereas delayed inflation will decrease coronary perfusion and reduce the amount of diastolic augmentation. Thus accurate timing is vital to the effective management of this device, and the occurrence of arrhythmias, particularly atrial fibrillation, will greatly decrease its efficiency.

Insertion of an IABP is not without complications. These include malposition, vascular damage, haemorrhage thrombosis, infection and confusion. The survival rate of patients who have had a balloon pump inserted following cardiac surgery is currently approximately 50%.

### Ventricular assist devices

Ventricular assist devices (including left ventricular, right ventricular and biventricular devices) can maintain an adequate pulmonary or systemic circulation in the presence of acute ventricular failure following cardiopulmonary bypass. The device is inserted in parallel to one or both ventricles, thus although the heart continues to beat the myocardial work is reduced enabling recovery to occur, or allowing time for a donor heart to be found. These devices may be described as tethered, where the patient is continuously connected via wires or tubes to an external component, or fully implanted, when the patient is free of all external components (excluding batteries).

Indications for the insertion of a ventricular assist device include mean arterial blood pressure less than 60 mmHg, cardiac index less than $1.8–2.0 \, L/min/m^2$, atrial pressure greater than 20 mmHg and a systemic vascular resistance greater than 2000 dyne/sec/cm$^{-5}$ (Scheld, 1997). Additional relative indications include oliguria, a mixed venous oxygen saturation less than 60%, a progressive acidosis or deteriorating blood gases. Absolute contraindications include multiorgan failure, septicaemia or irreversible brain damage.

The most common complications associated with the implantation of a ventricular assist device are bleeding, coagulopathy and infection.

### Reversal of heparin post-cardiopulmonary bypass

Once separation from cardiopulmonary bypass has been successfully achieved, and the circulation is stable, it is necessary to reverse the effects of the residual circulating heparin in order to prevent excessive postoperative bleeding. Currently, protamine sulphate, a sulphated polycationic peptide (highly positively charged) with a molecular weight of 4500 daltons is generally used. The ratio employed is 1–2 mg of protamine per 100 units of heparin given pre-bypass, or 0.8 mg of protamine per total dose of heparin given. When protamine is added to blood containing heparin, a stable bond is formed between the positively and negatively charged molecules. Heparin is no longer able to bind to antithrombin III, thus coagulation is normalized.

Protamine sulphate unfortunately may produce several undesirable side effects; these include systemic vasodilatation due to nitric oxide and histamine release, increased pulmonary vascular resistance, compromised ventricular function, thrombocytopenia, leukopenia and anaphylaxis. The severity of many of these effects is related to the rate of infusion (Wakefield *et al.*, 1996). Thus protamine should be administered over a period of at least 5 min to avoid potentially disastrous destabilization. Protamine also has a weak anticoagulant effect inhibiting platelet function, promoting fibrinolysis and therefore compromising clot structure (Carr and Carr, 1994). Thus the administration of an excessive dose of protamine is also undesirable.

## *Heparin rebound*

Although complete heparin neutralization may be achieved following protamine administration it is not uncommon for heparin to be detected in the plasma several hours following surgery. It is thought that the heparin is released from non-specific binding sites on plasma proteins. This heparin rebound does not, however, appear to be associated with an increased incidence of postoperative bleeding, and is probably not clinically significant (Martin *et al.*, 1992).

## Management of post-bypass coagulopathy

Cardiopulmonary bypass results in haemodilution of all the blood components including clotting factors and platelets. Indeed, in small adults it may be necessary to reduce the volume of the priming solution to limit this effect. Platelet function and numbers may be further compromised by the effects of heparin, protamine and exposure to the abnormal surface of the bypass circuitry. Furthermore, if for any reason the level of heparinization is inadequate, activation of the clotting cascade may occur and additional consumption of clotting factors will result. Fortunately careful attention to surgical haemostasis and the appropriate administration of protamine is generally all that is required to prevent excessive postoperative bleeding.

Certain patients are at an increased risk of bleeding post-bypass. These include patients who have undergone previous cardiac surgery, those with a known coagulopathy, those taking aspirin or other antiplatelet drugs, and those with evidence of local or systemic sepsis such as infective endocarditis. In these high risk cases it is essential to liaise with the haematology department to ensure a logical and structured approach to that particular patient's coagulopathy.

## Haematological management of postoperative bleeding

It is common practice in patients who are at an increased risk of postoperative haemorrhage to give a transfusion of platelets empirically immediately following the administration of protamine. Specific clotting factors may be also given at this stage in patients who have a known coagulopathy. If bleeding continues, regular assessment of the following is indicated: haemoglobin concentration, platelet count and function, heparin concentration, prothrombin time, activated partial thromboplastin time and fibrinogen level. Further blood, platelets, fresh frozen plasma and cryoprecipitate can then be given appropriately on the basis of the results of these tests.

The red cell requirement of these patients may be reduced by utilizing a cell saver in which blood collected from the surgical field is spun, washed and the red cells transfused back into the patient.

## Pharmacological management of postoperative bleeding

Following the administration of protamine, an assessment of the activated clotting time is performed. If this is prolonged and haemostasis is inadequate, an additional dose of protamine 50–100 mg is often given prior to any further assessment of coagulation. Several additional drugs are available to promote coagulation post-cardiopulmonary bypass. Aprotinin is probably the one used most commonly and will be discussed in more detail here.

### Aprotinin

Aprotinin is a non-specific serine protease inhibitor isolated from bovine lung. It inhibits plasmin and kallikrein and therefore inhibits the intrinsic clotting pathway, and plasmin-induced complement activation (Fig. 4.4) (Westaby, 1993). Aprotinin also acts to preserve platelet function These combined effects have been shown to reduce significantly the blood loss associated with cardiac surgery.

It is common for patients at an increased risk of bleeding post cardiopulmonary bypass to receive aprotinin, although its use in patients undergoing coronary revascularization remains controversial. Traditionally it was believed that to achieve the maximum benefit, aprotinin should be commenced in high doses ($2 \times 10^6$ KIU intravenously, $2 \times 10^6$ KIU in the priming solution and 500 000 KIU/hour) prior to skin incision. It is becoming increasingly apparent however that low dose regimes ($2 \times 10^6$ KIU in the prime) may have equal benefit. Commencement postoperatively in the patient who is bleeding excessively may also be useful.

**Table 4.4 Drugs used to promote haemostasis following cardiac surgery**

| Drug | Dose | Mechanism of action |
|------|------|---------------------|
| Protamine | 1–2 mg/100 units heparin | Binds with heparin and prevents activation of antithrombin III |
| Aprotinin | High dose 4 × 10⁶ KIU + 500 000 KIU/hour Low dose: 2 × 10⁶ KIU | Serine protease inhibitor; preserves platelets |
| Tranexamic acid | 0.5–3 g | Inhibits plasminogen activation and fibrinolysis |
| Desmopressin | 0.4 mcg/kg | Increases factor VIIIC and factor VIIIAg; promotes platelet aggregation |
| Ethamsylate | 12.5 mg/kg | Improves platelet adhesion; increases capillary vascular wall resistance |

Aprotinin therapy is associated with some potentially undesirable side effects. In the presence of heparin, aprotinin prolongs the activated clotting time. If the activated clotting time (ACT) is the only measure of the effectiveness of anticoagulation, it may then become uncertain as to whether the circulating heparin levels are adequate. Thus it is customary, in the presence of aprotinin, to maintain the ACT for more than 700 sec during cardiopulmonary bypass to incorporate an extra margin of safety. There is also some evidence that graft patency in coronary artery bypass patients is reduced in the presence of aprotinin, and that there may be a transient postoperative rise in creatinine, indicating an element of renal dysfunction in patients receiving aprotinin (Davis and Whittington, 1995). Occasionally aprotinin will provoke a severe allergic reaction; it is therefore advisable to give a test dose a few minutes prior to administering the full dose.

Other drugs which may be used in the promotion of haemostasis after cardiac surgery include tranexamic acid, desmopressin and ethamsylate (Table 4.4). With the possible exception of tranexamic acid, however, these drugs have not found a place in the routine management of patients' bleeding following cardiac surgery.

# References

Alkhulaifi A.M. (1997) Preconditioning the human heart. *Ann R Coll Surg Engl;* **79**(1): 49–54.

Bannan S., Danby A., Cowan D. *et al.* (1997) Low heparinisation with heparin bonded bypass circuits: is it a safe strategy? *Ann Thorac Surg;* **63**: 663–668.

Bashein G., Townes B.D., Nessly B.S. *et al.* (1990) A randomised study of carbon dioxide management during hypothermic cardiopulmonary bypass. *Anaesthesiology;* **72**: 7–15.

Buckberg G.D. (1995) Update on current techniques of myocardial protection. *Ann Thorac Surg;* **60**: 805–814.

Carr M.E. Jr and Carr S.L. (1994) At high heparin concentrations, protamine concentrations which reverse heparin anticoagulant effects are insufficient to reverse heparin anti-platelet effects. *Thromb Res;* **75**(6): 617–630.

Christakis G.T., Abel J.G. and Lichtenstein S.V. (1995) Neurological outcomes and cardiopulmonary temperature: A clinical review. *J Cardiac Surg;* **10**: 475–480.

Chung J.H., Gikakis N., Rao A.K. *et al.* (1996) Pericardial blood activates the extrinsic coagulation pathway during clinical cardiopulmonary bypass. *Circulation;* **93**: 2014–2018.

Cohen N.M., Damiano R.J. and Wechsler A.S. (1995) Is there an alternative to potassium arrest? *Ann Thorac Surg;* **60**: 858–863.

Davis R. and Whittington R. (1995) Aprotinin. A review of its pharmacology and therapeutic efficacy in reducing blood loss associated with cardiac surgery. *Drugs;* **49**(6): 954–983.

Gaer J.A., Shaw A., Wild R. *et al.* (1994) Effect of cardiopulmonary bypass on gastrointestinal perfusion and function. *Ann Thorac Surg;* **57**: 371–375.

Gold J.P., Charlson M.E., Williams-Russo P. *et al.* (1995) Improvement of outcomes after coronary artery bypass: a randomized trial comparing intraoperative high vs low mean arterial pressure. *J Thorac Cardiovasc Surg;* **110**: 1302–1314.

Gravlee G.P., Angert K.C., Tucker W.Y. *et al.* (1988) Early anticoagulation peak and rapid distribution after intravenous heparin. *Anaesthesiology;* **68**: 126–129.

Gravlee G.P., Davis R.F. and Utley J.R. (1993) In *Cardiopulmonary Bypass: Principles and Practice.* Williams and Wilkins, London.

Grocott H.P., Newman M.F., Croughwell N.D. *et al.* (1997) Continuous jugular venous versus nasopharyngeal temperature monitoring during hypothermic cardiopulmonary bypass for cardiac surgery. *J Clin Anesth;* **9**(4): 312–316.

Hartman G. (1997) Pro-con: mean arterial pressure should be maintained during cardiopulmonary bypass. *J Cardiothorac Vasc Anaesth*

Hett D.A. and Smith D.C. (1994) A survey of priming solutions used for cardiopulmonary bypass. *Perfusion;* **9:** 19–22.

Hindman B. (1995) Con: glucose priming solutions should not be used for cardiopulmonary bypass. *J Cardiothorac Vasc Anesth;* **9:** 605–607.

Hindman B.J., Dexter F., Smith T. *et al.* (1995) Pulsatile versus nonpulsatile flow. No difference in cerebral blood flow or metabolism during normothermic cardiopulmonary bypass in rabbits. *Anaesthesiology;* **82:** 241–250.

Indeglia R.A., Shea M.A., Forstrom *et al.* (1968) Influence of mechanical factors on erythrocyte sublethal damage. *Trans ASAIO,* **14,** 264–271.

Kirklin J.W. and Barratt-Boyes B.G. (1986) In *Cardiac Surgery.* John Wiley and Sons, Chichester, Chapter 45.

Knothe C.H., Boldt J., Zickmann B. *et al.* (1995) Influence of different flow modi during extracorporeal circulation on endothelial-derived vasoactive substances. *Perfusion;* **10:** 229–236.

Koska A.J., Romagnoli A. and Kramer W.G. (1981) Effect of cardiopulmonary bypass on fentanyl distribution and elimination. *Clin Pharmacol Ther;* **29:** 100–105.

Loomis C.W., Brunet D., Milne B. *et al.* (1986) Arterial isoflurane concentration and EEG burst suppression during cardiopulmonary bypass. *Clin Pharmacol Ther;* **40:** 304–313.

Martin P., Horkay F., Gupta N.K. *et al.* (1992) Heparin rebound phenomenon – much ado about nothing? *Blood Coagul Fibrinolysis;* **3**(2): 187–191.

Metz S. (1995) Pro: glucose priming solutions should be used for cardiopulmonary bypass. *J Cardiothorac Vasc Anesth;* **9:** 603–604.

Nanas J.N. and Moulopoulos S.D. (1994) Counterpulsation: historical background, technical improvements, haemodynamic and metabolic effects. *Cardiology;* **84:** 156–167.

Onoe M., Mori A., Watarida S. *et al.* (1994) The effect of pulsatile perfusion on cerebral blood flow during profound hypothermia with total circulatory arrest. *J Thorac Cardiovasc Surg;* **108:** 119–125.

Parault B.G. and Conrad S.A. (1991) The effect of extracorporeal circulation time and patient age on platelet retention during cardiopulmonary bypass: a comparison of roller and centrifugal pumps. *J Extra-Corpor Technol;* **23:** 34–38.

Philippou H., Davidson S.J., Mole T.M. *et al.* (1997) *Thrombosis and Haemostasis,* Suppl 15.

Scheld HH (1997) Mechanical support – benefits and risks. *Thorac Cardiovasc Surg;* **45:** 1–5.

Su H.B., Tseng C.C., Jenn C.T. *et al.* (1996) Changes of propofol levels in isolated cardiopulmonary bypass circuit. *Acta Anaesthesiol Sin;* **34**(1): 17–20.

Tamura M. and Tamura T. (1994) Non-invasive monitoring of brain oxygen sufficiency on cardiopulmonary bypass patients by near-infra-red spectrophotometry. *Med Biol Eng Comput;* **32:** S151–S156.

Tonz M., Mihaljevic T. and Pasic M. (1993) Is normothermic cardiopulmonary bypass associated with increased morbidity? *Helv Chir Acta;* **60**(3): 387–391.

Uretzky G., Landsburg G., Cohn D. *et al.* (1987) Analysis of microembolic particles origination in extracorporeal circuits. *Perfusion;* **2:** 9–17.

Wakefield T.W., Hantler C.B., Wrobleski S.K. *et al.* (1996) Effects of differing protamine reversal of heparin anticoagulation. *Surgery;* **119**(2): 123–128.

Watarida S., Mori A., Onoe M. *et al.* (1994) A clinical study on the effects of pulsatile cardiopulmonary bypass on the blood endotoxin level. *J Thorac Cardiovasc Surg;* **108:** 620–625.

Westaby S. (1993) Aprotinin in perspective. *Ann Thorac Surg;* **55**(4): 1033–1041.

Wheeldon D.R., Bethune D.W. and Gill R.D. (1990) Vortex pumping for routine cardiac surgery: A comparative study. *Perfusion;* **5:** 135–143.

# Chapter 5

# Early postoperative management of patients following cardiac surgery

## Transfer to the intensive care unit

Following cardiac surgery, patients usually spend a variable length of time either in an intensive care or high dependency unit. The transfer from theatre to this facility is a time of potential instability and the tendency by the theatre team to relax at the completion of surgery must be avoided. During transfer the level of monitoring is greatly reduced, ventilation is generally not automated and its effectiveness variable, and infusion pumps may be accidentally turned off, disconnected or suffer power failure. The patient will also continue to rewarm and may unexpectedly vasodilate or may be bleeding significantly, rendering him suddenly hypovolaemic. Similarly, any short-acting anaesthetic agents used during the procedure can wear off rapidly and allow the patient to regain consciousness. It is easy to appreciate that these factors may lead to highly undesirable swings in heart rate and blood pressure at a time when the rapid initiation of treatment may be difficult.

It is therefore important that systematic preparations are made prior to transfer. The maximum available level of monitoring available should be used, infusion pumps should be checked for syringes that are almost empty and limited battery life and replaced if necessary. Anaesthesia should be supplemented with further hypnotic agents and opiates as appropriate. Intravenous fluids should be primed, and vasoactive and anaesthetic drugs for bolus administration should be available for the transfer.

It is not generally necessary to clamp the chest drains during transfer; even if the pleura have been opened during surgery the development of a pneumothorax is unlikely in the presence of hand ventilation. If the chest drains are clamped it makes the detection of a sudden serious haemorrhage difficult to detect and the patient may rapidly develop cardiac tamponade.

When the patient arrives on the intensive care unit full monitoring and mechanical ventilation should be re-instituted as rapidly as possible and details of the operative procedure conveyed to the nurse and doctor subsequently caring for the patient. A plan should be formulated, with the aim of early extubation if appropriate in that particular patient.

During the early postoperative period the minimum monitoring acceptable consists of an electrocardiogram, invasive arterial pressure and right atrial pressure, arterial oxygen saturation, urine output, chest tube drainage and core and peripheral temperature measurement.

## Fluid replacement therapy

Appropriate fluid therapy post cardiac surgery is central to a successful outcome. Following cardiopulmonary bypass the extracellular fluid volume may increase by as much as 20–30% (Vlahakes *et al.*, 1994) due to the volume of the priming solution given, haemodilution and capillary leakage. The degree of this extracellular fluid overload increases with the increasing duration of bypass. Co-existent with this extracellular fluid overload, there may, however, be relative intravascular hypovolaemia. In the hours following surgery the patient will continue to warm up peripherally resulting in increasing vasodilatation, blood loss may be ongoing and the post-bypass diuresis may be marked. Thus, in order to maintain an adequate preload, administration of intravenous fluids may be essential. Constant vigilance is required in the assessment of volaemic status and appropriate fluid therapy should be maintained.

The patient's own washed red blood cells may be available for transfusion in the early postoperative period if a cell saver device was used during surgery. Also residual blood from the bypass circuitry may be re-infused into the patient towards the end of surgery. It should be remembered that although the latter forms a useful colloid, it will not increase the circulating haemoglobin concentration; it also contains heparin, necessitating reversal with supplemental protamine.

A commonly used regime prescribes post-operative fluid 1 ml/kg/hour of a crystalloid solution, e.g. dextrose saline to provide the maintenance requirements, plus colloid therapy (gelatin, hetastarch, blood and blood products) to replace blood and urinary losses and compensate for increasing vasodilatation. Moderate postoperative haemodilution has been shown to result in increased coronary blood flow, increased cardiac output and decreased left ventricular work, due to a reduction in blood viscosity and therefore afterload (Hagl *et al.*, 1977). In our institution, patients usually receive a blood transfusion if their haemoglobin level is less than 8 g/dl. Below this level the benefits described above are lost as the oxygen delivery to the myocardium is compromised. It must be remembered, however, that a patient should not receive a transfusion merely because his haemoglobin has fallen below a particular level; each patient should be assessed according to his risk of inadequate myocardial oxygenation, and transfused as appropriate. There is no evidence that mild to moderate anaemia contributes to peri-operative morbidity.

## Principles of chest drainage

All patients who have undergone cardiac surgery return from theatre with chest drains *in situ*. These are placed prior to wiring the sternum within the pericardial space and also in the pleural cavities, if the latter have been opened during surgery. As the thoracic cavity is closed, the drainage tubes are connected to an underwater seal and a negative pressure of approximately 5 kPa is applied thus helping to prevent the accumulation of fluid or air postoperatively. During transfer of the patient from theatre to the intensive care unit, the chest drain tubing is not clamped, but the bottles are transported at level lower than the patient's chest to avoid drainage of air and water into the pleural cavity. The drains are generally removed on the first postoperative day if drainage has been

50 ml or less in the preceding 4 hours. If this criterion has not been fulfilled they may be removed on the second postoperative day, or even later.

Despite the routine use of chest drains the incidence of echocardiographic pericardial effusion following cardiac surgery has been quoted as between 26 and 85%. Fortunately, this accumulation of fluid is generally clinically undetected and leads to cardiac tamponade in only 0.8–1.3% of cases (Smulders *et al.*, 1989).

## Postoperative bleeding

Because of the nature of cardiac surgery, the effects of cardiopulmonary bypass on the coagulation cascade and the use of high concentrations of heparin, patients undergoing cardiac surgery are at a significant risk of bleeding postoperatively. Bleeding may be described as severe (400 ml/hour), heavy (200–400 ml/hour) or moderate (200 ml/hour). It may be concealed, where it remains inside the chest as a pericardial or pleural effusion, or more commonly revealed, where it appears in the chest drain bottles. Continued haemorrhage may have a surgical cause, such as a slipped ligature or oozing suture line, or be due to a haematological problem such as disorders of the coagulation system, or residual heparin activity. It should be remembered that continued 'surgical' bleeding will eventually lead to platelet and clotting factor depletion and an associated coagulopathy.

If the patient is bleeding excessively postoperatively, a minimum of 4 units of blood should be requested at an early stage. A coagulation screen should be performed, including the thrombin time, prothrombin time, activated partial thromboplastin time, fibrinogen level, fibrin degradation products and a serum heparin concentration. A full blood count should also be carried out to assess the haemoglobin concentration and the platelet count. Remember that although the platelet count may appear adequate, platelet function is impaired by cardiopulmonary bypass potentially necessitating subsequent platelet transfusion. If any of the tests of coagulation are abnormal they should be corrected with infusion of the appropriate blood products. A variety of procoagulant drugs may also be used to control bleeding. These are discussed in more detail in Chapter 4.

If the bleeding continues or increases in the presence of a normal clotting screen, or signs of cardiac tamponade develop (increased filling pressure in the presence of systemic hypotension), the patient should be taken back to theatre and re-explored for a surgical source of the bleeding. Resternotomy under these circumstances is associated with a greatly increased morbidity and mortality. In one study (Unsworth-White *et al.*, 1995) the re-opening rate was 3.5%, and of these patients 22% died in hospital. This serves to emphasize the importance of meticulous haemostasis in the first instance. Occasionally severe bleeding renders the patient too unstable haemodynamically to be transferred back to the operating theatre for re-exploration. In this situation, the chest may be reopened in the intensive care unit in the understanding that the advantage of speed outweighs the disadvantages of poorer lighting, visualization, and an increased risk of infection. Adequate analgesia, anaesthesia and muscle relaxation must not be neglected for patients undergoing re-exploration on the intensive care unit.

# Rewarming post cardiac surgery

Following hypothermic cardiopulmonary, despite rewarming to a core temperature of 37°C prior to separation from bypass, the patient may remain peripherally cool for many hours. This may lead to significant core cooling, as cool blood from the peripheries mixes with the relatively warm blood from the central circulation. Other factors which contribute to delayed rewarming are the use of vasoconstrictors, non-humidified gases, the infusion of cold fluids and a prolonged period of haemostasis prior to closure of the chest. Thus it is not unusual for the patient to arrive on the intensive care unit with a core temperature of only 35°C. This may be limited by ensuring that gases are humidified and fluids warmed prior to infusion. Surface warming devices may also be useful, as may the judicious use of vasodilator drugs.

# Postoperative management of serum electrolytes

## Sodium

Major surgery results in a postoperative increase in the secretion of antidiuretic hormone (ADH) and aldosterone; this results in sodium and water retention and potassium excretion. The excretion of sodium via the kidneys often falls to less than 10 mmol/L resulting in an increase in total body sodium. There may be a paradoxical decrease in serum sodium levels as the conservation of water via ADH tends to be dominant. As cardiopulmonary bypass results in an increase in the extravascular fluid volume by as much as 30%, this additional fluid load is potentially undesirable. It is clear that vigorous administration of sodium-containing crystalloid fluids in the early postoperative period is inappropriate; 1 ml/kg/hour of dextrose saline represents an acceptable compromise.

## Potassium

In opposition to sodium and water, the renal excretion of potassium may increase to as much as 100 mmol/L. This, in conjunction with the diuresis that commonly occurs postoperatively and the long-term use of pre-operative diuretic therapy, may result in postoperative hypokalaemia. This can be severe and predispose to potentially hazardous cardiac arrhythmias. Severe hypokalaemia may manifest itself as a metabolic alkalosis with ECG changes including ST depression, T wave inversion and marked U waves. It is our policy therefore to maintain the serum potassium level between 4.5 and 5.0 mmol/L by infusing potassium chloride 10–20 mmol diluted in 50 ml of dextrose saline into a central vein over 30 min. Potassium should ideally be given via an infusion pump as rapid administration can result in asystole.

Hyperkalaemia occasionally occurs postoperatively if the usual aldosterone-induced excretion of potassium is prevented by renal failure. This, in conjunction with the use of large volumes of potassium-containing cardioplegia and a degree of haemolysis associated with cardiopulmonary bypass may result in life-threatening hyperkalaemia. A serum potassium level greater than 7.0 mmol/L is associated with peaked T waves, atrioventricular block and broadening QRS complexes. This should be rapidly treated with calcium chloride 10 mmol intravenously and 50 ml 50% dextrose with 10 units of soluble insulin, to prevent cardiac arrest. A rectally administered ion-exchange resin such as calcium resonium also promotes the subsequent excretion of potassium. Severe renal failure will ultimately require haemofiltration or haemodialysis to maintain the serum electrolytes within the normal range.

## Calcium

The serum calcium level decreases following cardiopulmonary bypass, principally as a result of haemodilution. This is usually transient, lasting less than 24 hours, and is not clinically significant in adults. Occasionally patients present for cardiac surgery with pre-existing hypocalcaemia. In this situation cardiopulmonary bypass will result in severe hypocalcaemia manifesting itself as hypotension, a low cardiac output, arrhythmias, a prolonged QT interval and T wave inversion. This can be treated with 5–10 ml of 10% calcium chloride intravenously, repeated, following laboratory assessment, as necessary. It is important to remember that calcium excretion will be impaired in the presence of renal failure and therefore any supplements should be administered with caution.

## Magnesium

The serum concentration of magnesium is also reduced following cardiopulmonary bypass, but in this case the reduction is greater than would be expected by haemodilution alone. The serum concentrations gradually return to the normal range during the first 10 postoperative days. This hypomagnesaemia is generally well tolerated, but in high-risk patients it predisposes to a reduced cardiac output, ventricular and supraventricular arrythmias and a prolonged requirement for ventilatory support (England *et al.,* 1992). These adverse effects are prevented by the intravenous infusion of 2 g magnesium sulphate diluted in 50 ml 5% dextrose over a period of 30 min.

# Postoperative acid/base management

Disturbances in acid/base balance are common following cardiac surgery. It is essential that a blood gas sample should be taken soon after arrival on the intensive care unit in order to detect any problems that have developed during transfer of the patient from theatre. The principal causes of abnormalities in acid/base balance are shown in Table 5.1.

As the patient is usually mechanically ventilated, any disturbances of acid/base balance with a respiratory aetiology can be rapidly corrected by adjusting the minute ventilation. In the case of a metabolic derangement, attention must be directed to the cause. A low cardiac output, hypovolaemia and poor peripheral perfusion is treated with fluids, inotropes and vasodilators. Hyperglycaemia and hypokalaemia should be corrected with insulin and potassium infusions respectively, and renal failure managed with normovolaemia, diuretics, dopamine and haemofiltration as necessary. Bleeding must be controlled, and any indication of sepsis should be managed vigorously with appropriate antibiotics and circulatory support if required. The use of sodium bicarbonate

**Table 5.1 Aetiology of acid/base disturbance following cardiac surgery**

| Acid/base disturbance | Aetiology | Effects |
|---|---|---|
| Metabolic acidosis | Poor cardiac output, poor systemic perfusion, poor renal function, sepsis, hyperglycaemia | Myocardial depression, decreased effectiveness of inotropes and vasopressors |
| Metabolic alkalosis | Hypokalaemia, severe hypovolaemia, massive transfusion | Arrhythmias, hypocalcaemia |
| Respiratory acidosis | Hypoventilation during transfer, inappropriate ventilator settings | Hypertension, arrhythmias, increased pulmonary vascular resistance |
| Respiratory alkalosis | Hyperventilation during transfer, inappropriate ventilator settings | Hypocalcaemia |

to correct an acute metabolic acidosis is generally not encouraged unless the pH is less than 7.1, or the base deficit is greater than −10.

Intravenous sodium bicarbonate is potentially deleterious in many ways:

- It increases the production of carbon dioxide which necessitates an increase in the minute ventilation
- It causes a shift of the haemoglobin dissociation curve to the left thus increasing the affinity of haemoglobin for oxygen and reducing oxygen delivery to the cells
- It provides a large sodium load to a patient in whom the total body sodium is already raised
- It is an exceedingly hypertonic solution and may cause local tissue necrosis if extravasation occurs
- It will inactivate adrenaline and dopamine and bind to calcium, thus the infusion line must be thoroughly flushed with saline prior to these drugs being given
- Hypokalaemia and hypocalcaemia may occur
- It can actually worsen the intracellular acidosis.

If the pH is less than 7.1, firstly attention must be paid to correcting the cause of the acidosis, then bicarbonate may be given according to the equation:

$$\text{Bicarbonate (mmol)} = \frac{\text{weight}}{3} \times \text{base deficit}$$

To prevent possible over-correction, half of this dose is given and then the blood gases are reassessed.

## Management of arrhythmias following cardiac surgery

Arrhythmias following cardiac surgery are not uncommon and may require rapid and effective treatment to prevent increasing morbidity and mortality. The principal causes of postoperative arrhythmias are shown in Table 5.2.

**Table 5.2 Common causes of arrhythmias following cardiac surgery**

| Mechanism of arrhythmia | Cause |
| --- | --- |
| Myocardial ischaemia | Hypotension, incomplete revascularization, early graft occlusion |
| Damage to the conducting system | Aortic valve replacement |
| Pre-existing arrhythmia | Long-standing atrial fibrillation in mitral valve disease |
| Electrolyte imbalance | Hypokalaemia, hyperkalaemia, hypomagnesaemia |
| Drugs | Digoxin, potassium chloride |
| Pacemaker failure | Disconnection of leads, pacing box turned off, loss of contact with the epicardium |
| Inadequate gas exchange | Hypoxia, hypercarbia |

It should be remembered at this stage that not all arrhythmias require treatment. It is almost invariably fruitless to spend time and effort trying to convert a patient back into sinus rhythm who has been in atrial fibrillation for many years. Many arrhythmias do, however, need prompt intervention. Any underlying predisposing factors should be corrected prior to the institution of specific anti-arrhythmic drugs. Thus hypotension, electrolyte imbalance, hypothermia and inadequate gas exchange should all be sought and corrected early. The practice of prescribing prophylactic beta-blockers to prevent postoperative arrhythmias after coronary artery surgery now appears to have fallen out of favour, as well constructed clinical trials have failed to demonstrate any benefit.

The therapeutic options available to control adverse arrhythmias may be divided into physical and pharmacological.

## Physical methods

Cardiac pacing can be used to increase the heart rate in the presence of a bradycardia, or by overpacing may be used to bring a tachycardia under control. As described in Chapter 4, pacing may be atrial, ventricular or dual chamber. It is desirable that the sequential nature of atrial and ventricular contraction is maintained, thus improving ventricular filling and atrioventricular valve function. This is best achieved with atrial or sequential pacing. Atrial pacing is, however, dependent upon an intact conducting system which is not always present. The optimal paced heart rate must be determined for each individual, but generally in an adult a rate of between 80 and 100 beats/min is appropriate. Rates much greater than 100 beats/min are undesirable as the myocardial oxygen consumption is unacceptably increased in the presence of a reduced coronary filling time. Heart rates at the lower end of this range allow satisfactory ventricular and coronary filling in patients with a non-compliant or 'stiff' ventricle.

Synchronized direct current cardioversion is a useful technique in the treatment of postoperative arrhythmias, in particular supraventricular tachycardia, ventricular tachycardia, atrial flutter and atrial fibrillation. A 50–360 Joules shock synchronized with the R wave of the electrocardiogram is delivered to the chest following correction of the predisposing factors discussed above, and institution of adequate anaesthesia.

### Pharmacological methods

Antidysrhythmic drugs commonly used following cardiopulmonary bypass include those classified by Vaughan Williams, cardiac glycosides and adenosine. These are shown in Table 5.3. It should be remembered that many postoperative

**Table 5.3 Commonly used antidysrhythmic drugs following cardiopulmonary bypass**

| Drug | Class* | Dose | Action | Comments |
|------|--------|------|--------|----------|
| Lignocaine | I | 1 mg/kg bolus dose 1–4 mg/min infusion | Membrane stabilizer, decreases $V_{max}$, increases threshold, decreases rate of spontaneous depolarization | Negative inotrope |
| Esmolol | II | 1 mg/kg bolus dose 50–200 mcg/kg/min | Decreases rate of spontaneous depolarization, decreased sympathetic activity | Short $T_{1/2}$, cardioselective |
| Labetalol | II | 5–50 mg bolus dose 15–120 mg/hour | Decreases rate of spontaneous depolarization, decreased sympathetic activity, alpha antagonist | Vasodilatation |
| Amiodarone | III | 300 mg bolus dose 900–1200 mg/ 24 hours | Prolongs duration of action potential, increased refractory period | Long $T_{1/2}$, multiple side effects |
| Verapamil | IV | 5–15 mg in divided doses | Decreased calcium entry into the cells | Must not give with beta-blockers |
| Digoxin | N/A | 0.5–1 mg in divided doses | Delays atrioventricular conduction, increased vagal activity | Toxicity is common |
| Adenosine | N/A | 3–12 mg rapid intravenous injection | Delays atrioventricular conduction | $T_{1/2}$ 8 sec, contraindicated in cardiac transplantation |

*Class refers to the Vaughan Williams classification

cardiac patients will be receiving infusions of pro-arrhythmogenic drugs such as dopamine or adrenaline. Often a reassessment of the continued need for these drugs, and possibly a reduction in the infusion rate help to bring the arrhythmia under control without the need for further agents.

An extensive discussion of all the antidysrhythmic agents available is beyond the scope of this book; however, the management of common dysrhythmias is discussed briefly below.

### Atrial flutter and atrial fibrillation

If hypotension is present, synchronized DC cardioversion is the treatment of choice. In the absence of hypotension, digoxin or amiodarone is used to control the atrial rate. Anticoagulation may be indicated to reduce the risk of embolization.

### Supraventricular tachycardia

If hypotension is present, synchronized DC cardioversion is appropriate. Otherwise vagal manoeuvres, such as carotid sinus massage, may rapidly restore sinus rhythm. If this fails adenosine can be given by rapid intravenous injection. Other effective drugs include beta-blockers, digoxin, amiodarone and verapamil (although the latter should not be given intravenously in a patient already receiving beta-blockers).

### Ventricular extrasystole and tachycardia

Similarly, if hypotension is present in association with ventricular tachycardia, synchronized DC cardioversion is the treatment of choice. Otherwise lignocaine or amiodarone are acceptable.

### Bradycardia

All bradycardias can be treated with cardiac pacing, atropine or isoprenaline. Isoprenaline may be contraindicated in patients with coronary artery disease because of the reduction in coronary perfusion secondary to the reduced diastolic pressure and increased heart rate. Cardiac pacing is preferable in this situation.

For the management of the pulseless rhythms, the reader is referred to readily available texts on cardiopulmonary resuscitation.

## Inotropic support following cardiac surgery

Patients undergoing cardiac surgery are, by the nature of their disease, at increased risk of postoperative myocardial dysfunction. This, coupled with the effects of cardiopulmonary bypass, and the difficulties in providing universally adequate myocardial protection results in the frequent need for postoperative inotropic support. It is vitally important, prior to commencing an inotropic agent, to ensure that the preload and afterload are first optimized. In the majority of patients, the left ventricular function determines overall cardiac performance, thus assessment of the left atrial pressure or the pulmonary capillary wedge pressure is useful to optimize left ventricular filling. Trans-oesophageal echocardiography, as described in Chapter 2 may similarly be used to assess volaemic status. If the left ventricular function is impaired, afterload reduction is beneficial prior to commencing inotropic therapy. If preload and afterload are optimized, and the cardiac output remains inadequate, then inotropic therapy should be commenced. The drugs commonly used are detailed in Table 4.1. In our institution, dopamine, dobutamine or dopexamine represent the first line agents of choice. If these do not provide an adequate increase in cardiac output, adrenaline and/or milrinone are added to the inotropic regimen. In the latter instance, noradrenaline may also be required to limit the sometimes excessive vasodilatation associated with this drug. It must be remembered that escalating inotropic therapy will require the measurement of cardiac output and the calculation of derived indices to guide subsequent clinical decision making.

## Dopamine

Dopamine has agonist action at alpha, beta and dopaminergic (DA) receptors. At lower doses its effect is predominantly at peripheral DA1 and DA2 receptors causing vasodilatation in the mesenteric circulation. In the kidney DA1 stimulation results in renal vasodilatation and naturesis DA2 stimulation has a synergistic effect on the DA1-modulated naturesis (Cheung and Barrington, 1996). At higher doses of dopamine, its sympathomimetic effects predominate. This results in a positive inotropic and chronotropic effect via cardiac beta receptors, and vasoconstriction via peripheral alpha receptors.

## Dobutamine

Dobutamine is a synthetic beta agonist with predominantly beta-1 cardiac effects. It has the disadvantage of causing a relatively marked tachycardia. Dobutamine may be administered via a peripheral vein.

## Dopexamine

Dopexamine is a synthetic drug structurally related to dopamine. It has marked agonist activity at beta-2 receptors and lesser activity at DA1, DA2 and beta-1 receptors. It also inhibits uptake 1. Thus dopexamine will reduce afterload via the beta-2 receptors, increase renal perfusion via the dopamine receptors and also have a mild indirect and direct inotropic effect (Fitton and Benfield, 1990). Dopexamine may also be given by infusion into a peripheral vein.

## Adrenaline

Adrenaline is a potent inotrope with both alpha and beta adrenergic effects. Beta-1 effects result in an increase in heart rate and cardiac output. Its activity at alpha receptors also augments the blood pressure and decreases renal perfusion by causing peripheral vasoconstriction. Beta-2 receptor activity results in bronchodilation.

## Noradrenaline

Noradrenaline has predominantly alpha effects resulting in peripheral vasoconstriction. It also has limited inotropic activity via cardiac beta-1 receptors. It should be remembered that peripheral vasoconstriction may be beneficial by improving coronary perfusion, but excessive increases in afterload will increase myocardial oxygen demand and predispose to further ventricular dysfunction.

## Milrinone

Milrinone is a second generation type III phosphodiesterase inhibitor. It acts by increasing intracellular cyclic adenosine monophosphate which results in a positive inotropic effect in the heart and vasodilatation in the periphery, including the pulmonary vasculature. Unlike the sympathomimetic agents, milrinone does not produce tolerance with prolonged use (Shipley *et al.*, 1996). As a significant proportion of the beneficial effect of milrinone is due to vasodilatation, as the infusion is weaned an angiotensin converting enzyme (ACE) inhibitor is often commenced in order to maintain this afterload reduction.

Generally, following the optimization of preload, afterload and inotropic support, the majority of patients can achieve a cardiac output and blood pressure adequate to maintain organ function and allow progressive recovery. However in 1–2% of patients one or both ventricles fail so severely that mechanical circulatory support is necessary. The use of mechanical circulatory support is a major undertaking; a successful outcome is dependent upon a multidisciplinary approach and good communication between all members of the team. The reader is referred to Chapter 4 for a more detailed discussion of the mechanical support of the failing heart.

# Renal support following cardiac surgery

Factors predisposing to coronary artery disease such as hypertension, hyperlipidaemia and diabetes also promote renovascular disease. Similarly, the effects of cardiac disease, i.e. poor cardiac output, will result in further renal dysfunction. Thus many patients presenting for cardiac surgery have pre-existing renal impairment. It is important to remember, at this point, that a normal pre-operative serum creatinine concentration does not preclude significant renal disease, as the level only begins to rise when the creatinine clearance has fallen to less than 30 ml/min.

During cardiopulmonary bypass, although it is now accepted that non-pulsatile flow is unlikely to be detrimental to renal function, further renal damage may occur as a result of ischaemia due to a low perfusion pressure, or haemolysis producing nephrotoxic free haemoglobin. The combination of these features places patients undergoing cardiac surgery at relatively high risk of postoperative renal failure. This in turn has an associated mortality of between 13% and 55% (Mangos *et al.*, 1995; Llopart *et al.*, 1997).

It is therefore important to pay strict attention to optimizing renal function throughout the peri-operative period. Pre-operatively, despite the often necessary use of diuretic therapy, extreme dehydration must be avoided. During cardiopulmonary bypass, the perfusion pressure should be maintained at a minimum of 50 mmHg, and higher in the presence of established renal failure. Postoperatively, attention should be directed at the maintenance of cardiac output, optimization of renal blood flow and avoiding the unnecessary use of nephrotoxic drugs.

## Nephroprotective drugs

Several drugs may be used peri-operatively to help to prevent renal damage. It should be remembered, however, that the maintenance of an adequate circulating volume and cardiac output are central to renal protection and attention should be paid to these factors prior to instituting drug therapy. Any drug that promotes a diuresis postoperatively will aid the recovery of normal renal function as it will limit renal tubular obstruction by cellular debris.

### Dopamine and dopexamine

As discussed earlier, dopamine binds to DA1 and DA2 receptors in the kidney, inducing renal vasodilatation with a resultant diuresis and naturesis. Although these effects aid fluid management, dopamine does not confer any specific protective effects upon the kidney. Dopexamine also binds to DA1 in the kidney, but it only has one-third of the potency of dopamine at these receptors (Broughton and Filcek, 1990) and therefore produces less renal vasodilatation than dopamine. Both dopamine and dopexamine do improve cardiac output, thus improving renal perfusion.

### Frusemide

Frusemide is a powerful loop diuretic acting upon the loop of Henle to increase sodium and water excretion. Frusemide also has vasodilatory properties acting to increase renal cortical blood flow and attenuate renal medullary hypoxia, thus it has a truly renoprotective effect (Brezis and Rosen, 1995). If a bolus dose of frusemide fails to produce a diuresis postoperatively, an infusion of 1–2 mg/min may be effective.

### Mannitol

Mannitol is a complex carbohydrate, which when given intravenously is freely filtered by the kidney and acts as an osmotic diuretic. Although the antioxidant effects of mannitol are probably overstated, it is likely that due to its osmotic effects it will result in a beneficial reduction in oedema of the renal tubular cells. However, in excessive quantities this osmotic diuresis may actually worsen medullary hypoxia. In moderate amounts, mannitol also tends to increase the circulating volume and decrease the haematocrit, both of which further improve renal perfusion.

### Urodilantin

Urodilantin is a polypeptide fragment of atrial naturetic peptide. It acts by dilating afferent renal arterioles and constricting efferent arterioles. This increases the pressure gradient across the glomeruli and promotes a diuresis and naturesis. Urodilantin may prove to be of benefit in the management of incipient oliguric renal failure post cardiac surgery and is increasingly used as another treatment option prior to the use of haemodialysis or haemofiltration.

Despite careful and appropriate management, up to 5% of patients post cardiac surgery will still go on to develop acute renal failure. Factors predisposing to postoperative renal failure include:

- Pre-operative renal failure
- Complex surgery, e.g. simultaneous coronary artery bypass grafting plus valvular surgery
- A long duration of operation, cardiopulmonary bypass time, or cross-clamp time
- Increasing age.

# Renal replacement therapy

The onset of acute postoperative renal failure is usually signalled by a period of oliguria, the passage of less than 30 ml of urine per hour for more than two consecutive hours. At this stage attention should be turned to ensuring that the urinary catheter is not blocked and that the cardiac output is not inadequate. Once these two possibilities have been excluded, the pharmacological options described above can be used to attempt to improve renal function. If oliguria persists, haemofiltration or dialysis may be necessary to prevent fluid overload, hyperkalaemia, acidosis or uraemia. Haemofiltration is generally preferable in this situation as it is a less complex technique and also takes longer to achieve the same effect. Thus patients are less likely to suffer haemodynamic instability secondary to major fluid shifts at this crucial time. It is also important at this stage to make sure that all nephrotoxic drugs are stopped, non-steroidal anti-inflamatory drugs must be avoided and aminoglycoside antibiotic toxicity prevented by closely monitoring plasma levels and adjusting the dose and dosage interval as appropriate.

## Haemofiltration

Continuous arteriovenous haemofiltration (CAVH) was originally developed in the 1970s to treat refractory oedema; however, its application to acute renal failure was rapidly realized. The patient's own blood pressure drives arterial blood through the haemofilter and then back to the patient via a venous line. This is analogous to the use of haemofiltration within the cardiopulmonary bypass circuit. The ultrafiltrate is collected separately and replaced with a suitable volume of isotonic fluid with an appropriate electrolyte composition. It is possible to remove 10–14 L of fluid per day using this method. However, the need for arterial access prompted the development of continuous venovenous filtration (CVVH).

CVVH requires the insertion of a large bore double lumen catheter. Blood is then propelled by means of a pump at a rate of 150–200 ml/min out of one lumen of the catheter, through the haemofilter and back to the patient via the other lumen. CVVH is the method most commonly used in the intensive care unit to treat postoperative acute renal failure. It is simple, venous access is usually gained easily and treatment can be started rapidly. Both of these techniques of haemofiltration, however, require anticoagulation, education of the nursing staff and close monitoring. Complications include haemorrhage, inadequate solute clearance, haemodynamic imbalance, inappropriate clearance of some drugs, and protein catabolism.

Both CAVH and CVVH may be combined with some of the advantages of haemodialysis by pumping dialysate in the opposing direction to the blood in the non-blood compartment of the haemofilter (continuous arteriovenous haemodiafiltration and continuous venovenous haemodiafiltration). This arrangement allows a better solute clearance in conjunction with smaller filtrate volumes.

### Dialysis

Dialysis, which is available for the management of renal failure on some intensive care units, may be divided into haemodialysis and peritoneal dialysis. Neither of these techniques is commonly used in adult patients in our unit, although peritoneal dialysis is often used in paediatric patients suffering from acute renal failure following cardiac surgery.

## Weaning from mechanical ventilation

Following cardiac surgery it is usual to undergo a period of mechanical ventilation. This period may be very short, or stretch into weeks. In either case it is necessary to set up a ventilator in the intensive care or recovery unit postoperatively. As a general principle, synchronized intermittent mandatory ventilation (SIMV) with pressure support is comfortable for the patient and allows early weaning if appropriate. Also SIMV will help prevent severe respiratory muscle wastage in patients who are ventilated for a considerable period of time.

Many patients who undergo cardiac surgery have been long-term cigarette smokers and are therefore at risk of significant pulmonary disease. In these patients pre-operative lung function tests including arterial blood gas analysis are useful to provide a baseline reference for subsequent management (see Chapter 1).

Factors leading to a delay in weaning from mechanical ventilation include:

- Pre-existing pulmonary disease
- Left ventricular failure
- Pneumonia
- Neurological damage
- Pneumothorax or pleural effusion
- Phrenic nerve injury associated with the use of topical slush
- Acute lung injury associated with cardiopulmonary bypass including acute respiratory distress syndrome (ARDS).

If ventilation is prolonged for more than 10 days, percutaneous tracheostomy may be performed in order to reduce dead space ventilation and facilitate weaning. When weaning is commenced, positive end expiratory pressure is reduced first followed by the inspired oxygen concentration, to 40% or less. Then the SIMV rate is reduced until the patient is receiving pressure support ventilation solely. It is common, in many units, for the patient to undergo a period of spontaneous ventilation via a T-piece prior to extubation. If this is used its duration must be limited to less than 30 min as deleterious basal atelectasis will rapidly occur.

# Acute lung injury following cardiopulmonary bypass

Cardiopulmonary bypass inevitably causes a degree of acute lung injury, although this is usually mild and not clinically significant. The changes are distinct from those due to the effects of anaesthesia, the site of the incision, the severity of postoperative pain and sputum retention. It is probable that this deterioration in lung function is due to an inflammatory response caused by the exposure of the circulating blood to the non-physiological surface of the bypass circuitry. Approximately 2% of patients suffer a severe injury and go on to develop acute respiratory distress syndrome (ARDS) which significantly delays their recovery. The acute lung injury is associated with a reduction in lung volume, a decrease in carbon monoxide transfer capacity, the loss of hypoxic pulmonary vasoconstriction and an increase in pulmonary vascular permeability. In combination these factors result in reduced pulmonary compliance, pulmonary oedema and deteriorating gas exchange. These patients require prolonged artificial ventilation and careful fluid management before the lungs can recover from the damage inflicted. Fortunately the mortality from ARDS related to cardiopulmonary bypass appears to be a great deal lower than that associated with sepsis or any of the other major causes of the syndrome.

# Postoperative analgesia

Although the pain arising from a median sternotomy is generally cited as being less severe than that from a lateral thoracotomy, it may still be substantial. Other potential sites of pain following cardiac surgery include the site of conduit harvest (arm or leg), the pharynx, neck, back, and groin if femoral cannulation has been used. Factors which are known to increase the intensity of pain associated with sternotomy include prolonged duration of operation, internal mammary artery harvest, milking and removal of the chest drains, and the use of endotracheal suction. The pain is generally more intense in the first 3 days (Bohachick and Eldridge, 1988) during which time opioid analgesia is required. This may be administered via the intravenous or epidural route. Intramuscular opiates are not an adequate method of analgesia following cardiac surgery. Effective acute pain management is essential particularly during the first 24 hours, not only for humanitarian reasons, but also as it aids mobility, promoting the early return of normal function and decreasing the incidence of development of chronic pain syndromes.

Intravenous opioids, e.g. morphine, are commonly prescribed following cardiac surgery. This can be in the form of a continuous infusion or as patient-controlled analgesia (PCA). It is important to note that with either of these methods peak receptor occupancy is not reached until at least 30 min following the intravenous injection of morphine, thus both must be initiated early to be maximally effective. Both methods provide good analgesia; however PCA has the advantage that the patient has control over his pain management. The disadvantages of PCA include the need for a certain level of understanding to use the system effectively, and the bolus dose and lockout time may not be appropriate for every patient. In addition, most commercially available disposable systems do not have the facility to programme a background infusion.

**Table 5.4 Advantages and disadvantages of epidural analgesia for cardiac surgery**

| Advantages | Disadvantages |
|---|---|
| Excellent analgesia | Full anticoagulation is necessary for cardiac surgery, therefore the incidence of epidural haematoma is likely to be increased |
| Facilitates early extubation and improves early postoperative lung function | May predispose to bradycardia and hypotension |
| Vasodilates the coronary arteries and reduces incidence of postoperative ischaemic events | Patient may be sedated for a prolonged period postoperatively thus making the detection of an epidural haematoma difficult |
| Reduces inflammatory response to cardiac surgery | Difficult to schedule as the epidural should be sited several hours, or preferably the day before surgery |
| Decreases the stress response to cardiac surgery | Has not been shown to improve outcome following cardiac surgery |

Epidural analgesia is being used increasingly to provide analgesia following cardiac surgery. Table 5.4 shows some of the advantages and disadvantages of this route of administration. It remains highly controversial as to whether the benefits of epidural analgesia following cardiac surgery outweigh the risks. It is, however, generally accepted that if an epidural is to be sited prior to cardiac surgery, this should be done the day prior to surgery to aid the detection and appropriate management of any immediate complications.

## Postoperative care of the fast-track patient

'Fast-track' cardiac surgery involves the early extubation and rapid transit through the intensive care unit of suitable low-risk patients. In order for this to be possible, patient selection must be undertaken with care (the reader is referred to Chapter 1 for further details). The surgery must be well planned and technically excellent, and the anaesthetic technique should include the use of volatile anaesthetic agents or ultra-short-acting opioids such as alfentanil or remifentanil. In addition the intensive care unit must be organized to facilitate early weaning and extubation. Of the patients deemed suitable for fast-track cardiac surgery, early extubation is not possible in 10–20%. This may be due to prolonged cardiopulmonary bypass associated with surgical difficulties, bleeding, or poor ventricular performance necessitating postoperative inotropic or mechanical support.

The benefits of early extubation include:

● Improved cardiac function, in particular improved diastolic compliance
● Reduced respiratory complications including a more rapid return of mucocillary function, less atelectasis and reduced nosocomial pneumonia
● Improved patient comfort
● Possibly decreased costs by better utilization of limited resources, although this has not yet been conclusively demonstrated.

When the fast-track patient is transferred to the intensive care unit following surgery the anaesthetist should provide the intensive care team with details of the patient's pre-operative characteristics, the anaesthetic technique, the operative findings and the post-bypass requirement for vasoactive and inotropic infusions. It is generally accepted that the use of vasoactive infusions or dopamine up to a dose of 5 mcg/kg/min does not preclude early extubation.

Synchronized intermittent mandatory ventilation is instituted as described above, and a propofol infusion commenced. If remifentanil was used in theatre this infusion is continued, otherwise postoperative analgesia is provided by a morphine infusion. A period of stabilization follows, during which the cardiovascular stability of the patient is assessed. Continued rewarming is facilitated, if necessary, with a warming blanket. Gas exchange, acid/base balance and chest tube drainage are also monitored. We aim to control the systolic blood pressure between 90 and 130 mmHg, treat any deleterious arrhythmias, achieve a core temperature greater than 36°C, maintain blood gases and acid/base status within acceptable limits and have a chest tube drainage of less than 50–75 ml/hour. When these preconditions are met, the propofol and remifentanil, if used, are stopped and the patient is allowed to wake up. It is important to note at this stage that although remifentanil is an extremely potent analgesic, its context sensitive half-life is only 3–5 min. It is therefore important to administer an alternative opiate such as morphine at least 30 min prior to discontinuing the remifentanil in order to prevent the occurrence of severe postoperative pain.

Once the patient is awake and able to obey commands, rapid weaning from ventilatory support occurs. Extubation is then performed by the nursing staff, when the patient is awake, able to communicate and comfortable. The respiratory rate should be within the normal range with a tidal volume sufficient to maintain adequate gas exchange. There should be no evidence of residual neuromuscular blockade.

This whole process generally takes between 1 and 4 hours. The vogue for extubating the cardiac patient in theatre immediately following surgery has generally fallen out of favour as rewarming may not be complete. In addition, factors such as postoperative bleeding and cerebrovascular injury, which may justifiably delay the weaning of ventilatory support, will not have been identified at this stage.

# References

Bohachick P. and Eldridge R. (1988) Chest pain after cardiac surgery. *Crit Care Nurse;* **8**(1): 16–22.

Brezis M. and Rosen S. (1995) Hypoxia of the renal medulla – its implications for disease. *N Engl J Med;* **332**(10): 647–655.

*British National Formulary* (1997) **33**: 67–80.

Broughton A.N. and Filcek S.A.L. (1990) Dopexamine hydrochloride. A combined vasodilator and positive inotrope with dopaminergic effects. *ITCM* November/ December

Cheung P.Y. and Barrington K.J. (1996) Renal dopamine receptors: mechanisms of action and developmental aspects. *Cardiovasc Res;* **31**(1): 2–6.

England M.R., Gordon G., Salem M. *et al.* (1992) Magnesium administration and dysrhythmias after cardiac surgery. A placebo-controlled, double-blind, randomised trial. *JAMA;* **268**(17): 2395–2402.

Fitton A. and Benfield P. (1990) Dopexamine hydrochloride. A review of its pharmacodynamic and pharmacokinetic properties and therapeutic potential in acute cardiac insufficiency. *Drugs;* **39**(2): 308–330.

Hagl S., Heimisch W., Meisner H. *et al.* (1977) The effect of haemodilution on regional myocardial function in the presence of coronary stenosis. *Basic Res Cardiol;* **72**: 344–364.

Llopart T., Lombardi R., Forselledo M. *et al.* (1997) Acute renal failure in open heart surgery. *Ren Fail;* **19**(2): 319–323.

Mangos G.J., Brown M.A., Chan W.Y. *et al.* (1995) Acute renal failure following cardiac surgery: incidence, outcomes and risk factors. *Aust NZ J Med;* **25**(4): 28409.

Shipley J.B., Tolman D. and Hastillo A. (1996) Milrinone: basic and clinical pharmacology and acute and chronic management. *Am J Med Sci;* **311**(6): 286–291.

Smulders Y.M., Wiepking M.E., Moulijn A.C. *et al.* (1989) How soon should drainage tubes be removed after cardiac operations? *Ann Thorac Surg;* **48**: 540–543.

Unsworth-White M.J., Herriot A., Valencia O. *et al.* (1995) Resternotomy for bleeding after cardiac operation: a marker for increased morbidity and mortality. *Ann Thorac Surg;* **59**: 664–667.

Vlahakes G.J., Lemmer J.H., Behrendt D.M. *et al.* (1994) Postoperative management. In *Handbook of Patient Care in Cardiac Surgery,* Little, Brown, Boston, pp. 62–104.

# Pre-operative assessment – thoracic anaesthesia

## Introduction

Lung resection is commonly undertaken in developed countries in an attempt to cure lung cancer. Lobectomy and pneumonectomy are the most frequently performed operations but occasionally bilobectomy is carried out on the right and, less frequently, sleeve resection of a bronchus is combined with lobectomy.

Lung resection inevitably leads to loss of functioning lung tissue except on the rare occasion when the disease process has already destroyed the lobe or lung to be removed. The assessment of pre-operative lung function is of great importance in these patients if they are to survive surgery at a reasonable risk and have a satisfactory quality of life postoperatively. The most recently available national figures show a peri-operative mortality of approximately 3% for lobectomy and 8% for pneumonectomy (Table 6.1), although mortality for pneumonectomy is usually in the region of 6% nationally.

This chapter concentrates on the assessment of the lung resection candidate but it is important to emphasize that patients presenting for other forms of thoracic surgery may have greater impairment of lung function. Those undergoing lung volume reduction surgery, lung biopsy and lung transplantation may all have very poor lung function. Pre-operative lung function will require assessment in those undergoing oesophageal surgery. It is also of great concern in patients with cystic fibrosis scheduled for what would, in fit patients, be relatively minor procedures such as Hickman line insertion or pleurodesis for pneumothorax. Pre-operative assessment for procedures other than lung resection is covered in Chapter 8.

**Table 6.1 Mortality rates – resection of primary lung tumours**

| Operation | No. | Deaths | % Mortality |
|---|---|---|---|
| Pneumonectomy | 902 | 74 | 8 |
| Lobectomy | 1795 | 52 | 2.9 |
| Segmentectomy/wedge resection | 205 | 1 | 0.5 |
| Chest wall resection with any lung resection | 66 | 6 | 9.1 |
| Exploratory thoracotomy (no resection) | 336 | 16 | 4.8 |

UK Thoracic Surgical Register 1995–1996 (returns from 37 of 41 NHS units)

## General anaesthetic assessment

The patient presenting for lung resection will have been fully evaluated by the appropriate medical and surgical teams prior to surgery. The anaesthetist should briefly review their findings and, where necessary, investigate factors specifically relevant to anaesthesia (see also Chapter 1). A proforma similar to Table 1.1 will aid collation of relevant data. Major pre-existing disease, such as diabetes mellitus, is noted and drug therapy continued where appropriate. In the case of respiratory disease it is important to continue bronchodilator therapy up to and including the morning of operation. Many of these patients will also have pre-existing cardiovascular disease; antianginal therapy and antihypertensive medication should be continued as described in Chapter 1. Aspirin and non-steroidal anti-inflammatory drugs are discontinued at least 1 week prior to surgery.

The anaesthetist should also note, at this stage, any features which suggest difficult tracheal intubation as these problems are often compounded when bulky and cumbersome endobronchial tubes have to be placed. The site and position of the trachea should also be ascertained clinically and on a chest X-ray because of its relevance to endobronchial tube placement. For similar reasons, distortion of the main bronchi evident on a chest X-ray or CT scan will have relevance to endobronchial intubation. It is also useful to record the height and weight of the patient at this time and note physical features such as a short neck and abnormal body build which may all influence the choice and size of endobronchial tube to be used intra-operatively. Abnormalities of the cervical, thoracic and lumbar spine should be noted as they may make positioning of the patient in the lateral thoracotomy position difficult or dangerous. Hyperextension of the neck in the supine position for bronchoscopy or mediastinoscopy is also particularly hazardous in the presence of an unstable cervical spine.

An intercostal drain may be *in situ* in certain circumstances, although this is unlikely in patients presenting for first-time lung cancer surgery. If a drain is present the quantity of blood, pus or air draining should be noted. A large air leak may cause difficulties during positive pressure ventilation (see management of bronchopleural fistula, Chapter 8) and an empyema in communication with the airway can cause contamination of the contralateral lung, especially in the lateral thoracotomy position. Both these problems can be overcome with endobronchial intubation and isolation of the affected lung.

## General investigations

As for cardiac surgery all patients require a recent chest X-ray, an ECG, full blood count and urea and electrolyte measurements, liver function tests and pre-operative blood crossmatch. We usually prepare two units of blood or packed cells for a routine lung resection. As detailed below baseline lung function tests are required in all patients but individuals may warrant more extensive tests of cardiorespiratory function.

The major part of the pre-operative assessment will, of necessity, focus on the cardiovascular and respiratory systems and this is discussed in more detail below.

# Assessment of the cardiovascular system

Many patients presenting for lung resection will be relatively elderly and life-long smokers. Not surprisingly morbidity and mortality from cardiovascular disease is common following thoracic surgery (see Table 6.2) and therefore it must be recognized pre-operatively in order to initiate or optimize treatment and estimate the risk of surgery. The Goldman Multifactorial Risk Index (Tables 6.3 and 6.4) is often quoted as a means of quantifying the cardiovascular risk associated with non-cardiac surgery. It is by no means a perfect scoring system. In particular it does not assign a score to hypertensive patients. It has been confirmed by other studies to have a high specificity but low sensitivity. In

**Table 6.2 Causes of death following lung resection for primary lung tumours**

| | Numbers of patients | |
|---|---|---|
| | Lobectomy | Pneumonectomy |
| MI/CCF/Cardiac arrest | 3 | 1 |
| Pulmonary embolus | 1 | 1 |
| Respiratory failure | 5 | 2 |
| Renal failure | 3 | – |
| Multi-organ failure | 1 | – |
| Other | 2 | 1 |

MI, myocardial infarction; CCF, congestive cardiac failure
Above figures include 20 resection deaths over a 4-year period. These are:
Pneumonectomy (1° malignant): 5 deaths of 137 cases (3.6% mortality)
Lobectomy (1° malignant): 15 deaths of 225 cases (4.4% mortality)
(Royal Brompton Hospital 1990–1994)

**Table 6.3 Multifactorial risk index – non-cardiac surgery**

| Risk factor | Points |
|---|---|
| History | |
| Myocardial infarction within 6 months | 10 |
| Age >70 years | 5 |
| Physical examination | |
| S3 gallop rhythm or raised jugular venous pressure | 11 |
| Important aortic stenosis | 3 |
| Electrocardiogram | |
| Rhythm other than sinus or sinus plus atrial premature beats on last pre-op ECG | 7 |
| Ventricular ectopic beats (>5 per min) | 7 |
| Poor general medical status* | 3 |
| Intraperitoneal, intrathoracic or aortic surgery | 3 |
| Emergency operation | 3 |

*Includes $PaO_2$ <8 kPa; $PaCO_2$ >6.7 kPa; creatinine >260 mmol/litre
(Goldman et al., 1977)

**Table 6.4 Performance of Goldman risk index in practice**

| Points | Life-threatening complications (%) | Cardiac deaths (%) |
|---|---|---|
| 0–5 | 0.7 | 0.2 |
| 6–12 | 5 | 2 |
| 13–25 | 11 | 2 |
| 26 or more | 20 | 56 |

(Goldman, 1977 and 1995)

practice this means that high scoring patients are likely to be high risk but not all high-risk patients are identified. At least it is a way of assessing individual patients objectively and it will be noted that patients above 70 years of age undergoing thoracic surgery immediately accrue 8 points on this scoring system. The American College of Cardiology and the American Heart Association have recently published extensive guidelines for peri-operative cardiovascular evaluation for non-cardiac surgery (see references). Clinical predictors of increased

**Table 6.5 Clinical predictors of increased peri-operative cardiovascular risk (myocardial infarction, congestive heart failure, death)**

**Major**
Unstable coronary syndromes
   Recent myocardial infarction* with evidence of important ischaemic risk by clinical symptoms or non-invasive study
   Unstable or severe angina (Canadian Class III or IV)**

Decompensated congestive heart failure

Significant arrhythmias
   High-grade atrioventricular block
   Symptomatic ventricular arrhythmias in the presence of underlying heart disease
   Supraventricular arrhythmias with uncontrolled ventricular rate

Severe valvular disease

**Intermediate**
Mild angina pectoris (Canadian Class I or II)
Prior myocardial infarction by history or pathological Q waves
Compensated or prior congestive heart failure
Diabetes mellitus

**Minor**
Advanced age
Abnormal ECG (left ventricular hypertrophy, left bundle branch block, ST–T abnormalities)
Rhythm other than sinus (e.g. atrial fibrillation)
Low functional capacity (e.g. inability to climb one flight of stairs with a bag of groceries)
History of stroke
Uncontrolled systemic hypertension

*Recent MI defined as greater than 7 days but less than or equal to 1 month (30 days)
**May include 'stable' angina in patients who are unusually sedentary
From American College of Cardiology/American Heart Association guidelines for perioperative cardiovascular evaluation for noncardiac surgery. (1996) *Circulation;* **93:** 1278–1317

peri-operative cardiovascular risk estimated in this review are detailed in Table 6.5. Intra-thoracic surgery is considered to be an intermediate (as opposed to high or low) risk for cardiac death and non-fatal myocardial infarction by these authors. Mangano (1990), on the other hand, has previously stated that patients undergoing thoracic or upper abdominal surgery have a 2–3-fold higher risk of peri-operative cardiac complications.

Cardiac dysfunction is particularly relevant following pneumonectomy where the whole of the cardiac output has to pass through one remaining lung. Significant pulmonary hypertension and right heart failure due to lung disease is likely to preclude major lung resection but lesser degrees of pulmonary vascular disease may be tolerated. In a widely quoted study (Table 6.6) Baier (1980)

**Table 6.6 Pulmonary vascular criteria for non-resectability**

| | |
|---|---|
| Mean PAP at rest | >22–30 mmHg |
| Mean PAP at rest on balloon occlusion | >26–32 mmHg |
| Mean PAP during exercise on balloon occlusion | >35 mmHg |
| Systemic $PaO_2$ during exercise on balloon occlusion | <6.0 kPa |

PAP, pulmonary artery pressure
Summary from Baier (1980) of criteria based on the assessment of pulmonary vascular function (see text) which has been associated with an increased mortality after pulmonary resection

attempted to quantify the risk of pulmonary vascular disease and lung resection by measuring pulmonary artery pressure in the catheter laboratory pre-operatively. This was done at rest, during exercise and with balloon occlusion of the pulmonary artery on the side of planned pneumonectomy. Whilst an interesting study it must be remembered that surgical techniques and the treatment of cardiovascular disease have improved since this was carried out in 1980. This type of complex and expensive investigation, therefore, has not been adopted clinically and remains a research tool. Cardiorespiratory function can be investigated more easily, although less specifically, by exercise testing and to a certain extent by the measurement of maximum breathing capacity. The merits of these tests are discussed below.

## Assessment of the respiratory system

### Clinical history

The clinical history is of great importance in the initial diagnosis of chest diseases. It will also be of interest to the anaesthetist but of less importance in the pre-operative assessment of the patient already admitted to hospital for lung resection. Symptoms of dyspnoea, cough and haemoptysis are relevant to the conduct of anaesthesia, however.

Dyspnoea is extremely subjective and difficult to quantify by direct questioning. An active patient with little or no exercise limitation due to breathlessness is likely to tolerate lung resection and even pneumonectomy without problems. This category of patient will only require pre-operative arterial blood gas analysis and baseline bedside spirometry. A patient whose exercise capacity is severely limited (e.g. only able to climb one flight of stairs without stopping) may not tolerate lung resection and will require careful pulmonary evaluation. Patients who are significantly breathless at rest are unlikely to tolerate any significant lung resection for the treatment of lung cancer but may present for other types of procedure such as lung volume reduction and lung biopsy.

Many patients with lung cancer have a cough. For the patient deemed operable this is rarely a problem. A productive cough with infected sputum may be evidence of infection beyond a tumour or may be a sign of generalized pulmonary infection in a smoker with chronic obstructive airways disease. In the presence of a generalized chest infection pre-operative physiotherapy and appropriate antibiotic therapy is indicated.

Minor haemoptysis is not usually worrying in the cancer patient but may forewarn of intra-operative bleeding which will be contained by the use of a double lumen endobronchial tube. Major haemoptysis is uncommon with operable malignant lesions but can, very rarely, necessitate emergency lung resection, particularly if the bleeding is exacerbated by bronchoscopic biopsy. Haemoptysis due to cavitating tuberculosis, aspergilloma and arteriovenous malformations is much more worrying and potentially difficult to deal with surgically.

## Physical examination

The physical examination will, of necessity, be brief and aimed mainly at the points of general anaesthetic interest discussed above. In addition to these points auscultation of the chest may reveal further information, such as the presence of wheeze, which will aid the interpretation of the pre-operative chest X-ray and lung function tests.

## Investigations

### Chest X-ray

Inspection of a postero-anterior (PA) and lateral chest X-ray will demonstrate the site of any localized lesion and its relationship to the hilum, mediastinum and chest wall. These X-rays, together with the CT scan, may corroborate the side of planned surgery and therefore should be on display in the anaesthetic room prior to induction of anaesthesia.

As previously discussed, the direction, shape and diameter of the trachea and main bronchi can often be determined from the pre-operative chest X-ray and this may alert the anaesthetist to potential problems with endobronchial intubation. This is another reason to display the X-rays in the anaesthetic room.

Apart from specific lesions, generalized lung pathology, related to cardiac or concomitant pulmonary disease, should be noted. Almost invariably more than one imaging technique is required to assess the extent and operability of lung cancer. These are discussed below.

## Computed tomography (CT scan)

CT scanning and faster scanning techniques (Imatron) are now an established method of demonstrating lesions within the thorax, some of which cannot be readily demonstrated by conventional radiology. CT scanning, with contrast enhancement, is used to identify the site, size and possible extension of intrathoracic tumours originating in the lungs and hilum. Patients with primary lung cancer are accepted for surgery, provided there are no distant metastases and if there is no evidence of nodal spread on a good quality CT scan. Those with hilar and mediastinal lymphadenopathy evident on a scan will need to undergo mediastinoscopy and biopsy of these nodes. This is because previous infective conditions and reactive hyperplasia of the nodes can cause appearances identical to that of malignant enlargement. Should the nodes be invaded with tumour the patient is unlikely to be curable by lung resection.

We routinely extend our CT scanning to include the brain, liver and adrenals in a search for metastatic disease. Many clinicians reserve brain CT for those patients with relevant neurological complications.

## Magnetic resonance imaging (MRI)

Magnetic resonance imaging techniques have not proved superior to CT scanning for the investigation of intrathoracic pathology. MRI may be useful, however, for the delineation of vascular structures and the imaging of neural tumours.

## Positron emission tomography (PET scan)

2-[f-18] fluoro-2-deoxy-D-glucose (FDG) has an increased uptake in malignant cells. Positron emission tomography using FDG is a non-invasive imaging modality which has been found to be highly accurate in differentiating benign from malignant solitary pulmonary nodules and lung lesions. It may also be useful in tracking down sites of tumour, although this is still relatively experimental.

## Other scanning techniques

### Bone scan

Radioisotope scanning techniques are used in patients with lung cancer to detect bony secondaries. We scan those patients who have bone pain or significant weight loss. Bone scans have a high false-positive rate due to Paget's disease, arthritis, healing fractures, renal disease and hyperparathyroidism. If an isolated bony lesion is identified, therefore, it should be biopsied under radiological control before the patient is denied surgery.

### Liver scan

A CT scan may show liver abnormalities but if this is not diagnostic a liver ultrasound can differentiate between cystic and solid lesions. If there is real doubt concerning the nature of a lesion in the liver a biopsy can be undertaken under CT or ultrasound control.

## Lung function tests

### Arterial blood gas analysis

We routinely measure arterial blood gas values with the patient breathing room air pre-operatively. This provides a useful baseline to compare with post-operatively. Arterial hypoxaemia is generally considered to be a poor indicator of risk for lung resection, although Nunn et al. (1988) found this to be the best predictor of the use of postoperative ventilation in patients with severe chronic obstructive airways disease undergoing general surgery. In thoracic surgery the portion of lung to be removed may be contributing to a physiological shunt with persistent blood flow but little or no ventilation, although this is offset to some extent by the compensatory mechanism of hypoxic pulmonary vasoconstriction. In marginal cases this can be investigated by ventilation–perfusion scanning techniques. It is also important to remember that arterial oxygen tension drops as part of the ageing process, the lower limit for normal in the 70–79 years age group being 9 kPa but just above 10 kPa in the 50–59 years age range.

An arterial carbon dioxide level greater than 6 kPa is held to represent increased peri-operative risk of pulmonary complications and mortality. This level of hypercapnia is not an absolute contraindication to lung resection, however, and has to be interpreted in conjunction with other lung function tests.

### Bedside spirometry

As discussed above relatively fit patients with good exercise tolerance only require baseline measurements of forced vital capacity (FVC) and forced expired volume in 1 sec ($FEV_1$). These can be carried out at the bedside or in the outpatient clinic. If the $FEV_1$ is above 2 L and the FVC above 50% of predicted values the patient is likely to tolerate pneumonectomy and no further lung function testing will be required (Crapo, 1994). If values fall significantly below these figures, particularly if $FEV_1$ approaches 1 L, it is preferable to carry out formal lung function testing in the laboratory.

## Laboratory lung function testing

Formal pulmonary function testing allows accurate measurement of static and dynamic lung volumes and other indices of lung function such as gas transfer. These measurements are carried out before and after bronchodilator therapy and results should be compared with normal values related to age, sex, size and ethnic origin. A variety of indices have pointed to increased risk after lung resection (Table 6.7) but time and again the literature refers to minimum values for $FEV_1$ in relation to different types of lung resection. It appears that an $FEV_1$ of 800–1000 ml is required to produce an effective cough to aid clearance of secretions. It is considered that, in a patient of average size, an $FEV_1$ of 1 L is required for that patient to have a reasonable chance of surviving pneumonectomy without a significant risk of respiratory failure in the postoperative period. Some authors consider that a predicted postoperative $FEV_1$ of 800–1000 ml is the cut-off point for pneumonectomy. This was previously calculated on the basis of functional losses (in relation to pre-operative values) of 25% for lobectomy or 33% for pneumonectomy. Postoperative function will, however, depend on the state of lung tissue to be resected and therefore more accurate predictions can be made using pre-operative radioisotope ventilation–perfusion scanning tech-

**Table 6.7 Summary of criteria widely considered to indicate a greater-than-normal risk of morbidity or mortality following lung resection**

| | |
|---|---|
| FVC | <50% predicted |
| $FEV_1$ | <2.0 L or 50% predicted |
| MBC | <50% predicted |
| $PaCO_2$ | >6.0 kPa |
| RV/TLC | <50% predicted |
| $T_LCO$ | <50% predicted |

RV/TLC, ratio of residual volume to total lung capacity; $T_LCO$, gas transfer; other abbreviations as text

niques. Radiospirometry with inhaled $^{133}Xe$ is used to assess ventilation and this can be matched to a radioisotope scan of lung perfusion following the intravenous injection of macro-aggregates radiolabelled with technetium.

In patients with a marginal $FEV_1$ the measurement of maximum breathing capacity (MBC) or formal exercise testing may yield additional information as a means of identifying patients at risk of pulmonary insufficiency post resection.

### Maximum breathing capacity

Maximum breathing capacity (MBC) is obtained by a period of voluntary hyperventilation through a low resistance circuit. This is usually for a period of 15 sec and minute volume is extrapolated from this. Motivation and sustainable muscle strength contribute to successful performance of this test. As these factors are important in the postoperative recovery period, it is not surprising that the test is reasonably predictive of morbidity and mortality. Patients with an MBC of less than 50% of the predicted value are at increased risk of hospital mortality. A figure of 40 or 20 L/min/m$^2$ body surface area, corresponding to an $FEV_1$ of approximately 1 L after resection, are widely regarded as a threshold below which the risks of respiratory failure following pulmonary resection are unacceptable.

### Exercise testing

In an attempt to improve pre-operative risk assessment several studies have been undertaken to evaluate cardiopulmonary exercise testing. It appears from some of these studies that when patients have a peak oxygen uptake ($\dot{V}O_2$), during exercise, of less than 15 ml/kg/min, the risk of postoperative complications increases.

As oxygen uptake is related to cardiac output it would not be surprising if peak oxygen uptake correlated with cardiac complications post lung resection. On the other hand, it is difficult to see how $\dot{V}O_2$ could predict pulmonary complications, such as sputum retention and lobar collapse, postoperatively. Some studies have found no predictive value of exercise testing in relation to the risk of lung resection and therefore the results of these tests should continue to be interpreted with caution.

## Summary – assessment of the lung resection candidate

The assessment of the lung resection patient is concentrated on the cardiovascular and respiratory systems. Minimum levels of lung function for various degrees of pulmonary resection are summarized in Table 6.8 and a practical approach to pre-operative assessment is summarized in the flow diagram in Fig. 6.1. In general, an holistic approach is sensible and no patient should be denied surgery on the basis of a single lung function test.

Despite the sophistication of currently available specialized tests, it is likely that, in patients with poor lung function, the final decision regarding surgery will

**Table 6.8 Suggested whole lung pulmonary function criteria for lung resection**

| Test | Pneumonectomy | Lobectomy | Wedge or segment |
| --- | --- | --- | --- |
| MBC (% predicted) | >55 | >40 | >35 |
| $FEV_1$ (L) | >2* | >1 | >0.6 |
| $FEV_1$ (% predicted) | >55 | 40–50 | >35–40 |

*Accepting this value as absolute lower limit for pneumonectomy may be unduly pessimistic (see also Fig. 6.1)
MBC, maximum breathing capacity; $FEV_1$, forced expiratory volume in 1 sec
(Adapted from Thomas *et al.*, 1995)

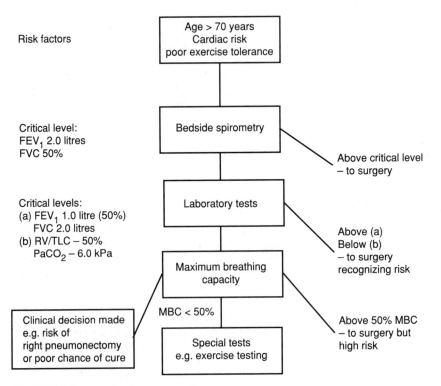

**Fig. 6.1** Risk factors and pulmonary resection

be made by the surgeon following routine laboratory pulmonary function testing. Surgery offers the only chance of long-term survival for non-small cell lung cancer and therefore, after discussion with the patient and close relatives, a relatively high element of risk may be acceptable if there is good chance of surgical success as ascertained by pre-operative staging. On the other hand, if the patient is elderly, has significant cardiac disease and requires an extensive lung resection (such as right pneumonectomy) it may be decided the risk is prohibitive and that palliative radiotherapy is preferable.

## Pre-operative preparation

Fit patients require little pre-operative preparation but they should be instructed by a physiotherapist so that they are familiar with the breathing exercises and coughing which will be required postoperatively.

Smokers should be encouraged to stop pre-operatively. Cessation of smoking is followed by a decrease in the volume of mucus hypersecretion and airway reactivity as well as improved mucociliary transport. These beneficial effects may lessen the incidence of postoperative atelectasis and infection but take approximately 2–4 weeks to develop. The short-term effects of stopping smoking (48–72 hours) may be associated with increased secretions and hyperactive airways. In this group there will, however, be a decrease of carboxyhaemoglobin content and better oxygen delivery to the tissues.

More attention should be given to the preparation of patients with poor lung function, particularly if there is a treatable component to their disease such as reversible airway obstruction, infected sputum or a source of re-infection in the sinuses or teeth.

Drugs which can be used to relieve bronchospasm include sympathomimetic agents, oral theophylline derivatives, ipratropium bromide (Atrovent) and inhaled corticosteroids such as beclomethasone dipropionate. For patients not already on one of these agents, we tend to use the sympathomimetic agent salbutamol and combine this with the antimuscarinic agent ipratropium bromide, where necessary. These can be given by aerosol or nebulizer, but the latter route is preferable in the pre-operative period.

Patients with lung cancer and a superimposed chest infection may well require antibiotic treatment at home prior to admission to hospital. Those with a chronic pulmonary infection may need admitting to hospital for several days pre-operatively so that sputum can be cultured, appropriate antibiotics given and physiotherapy commenced. This scenario, uncommon in the average patient with lung cancer, is routine in the few patients with bronchiectasis presenting for lung resection.

### Pre-medication

We no longer prescribe 'heavy' sedative pre-medication for patients about to undergo lung resection. After a sympathetic explanation of peri-operative events and a discussion of analgesic techniques to be used postoperatively (see Chapter 9) we find most patients are calm and satisfactorily sedated following the administration of temazepam (10–20 mg) given orally 1–2 hours prior to surgery. We also encourage oral hydration to within 2–4 hours of surgery unless there is a specific contraindication. Most of our patients are allowed a cup of tea on the morning of surgery.

We do not prescribe antisialogogues pre-operatively but prefer to give the anticholinergic glycopyrronium bromide (glycopyrrolate) intravenously during surgery if hypersecretion becomes a problem.

### Ancillary drug therapy

As discussed above all relevant medication is continued up to the time of surgery. Diabetics may need stabilization on a sliding scale of intravenous insulin pre-operatively, but this is unusual.

The vast majority of patients are given low molecular weight heparin subcutaneously, starting on the morning of operation and continuing into the postoperative period. Our practice for thromboprophylaxis is described in more detail in Chapter 9.

Antibiotic prophylaxis is started immediately after the induction of anaesthesia and continued for 24 hours. We currently give a first generation cephalosporin (cephazolin) intravenously, unless this is contraindicated or there is bacteriological evidence that a different drug is more appropriate.

Antibiotic prophylaxis in the peri-operative period remains controversial, however, and many different regimes are used.

We do not administer anti-arrhythmic drugs prophylactically, but obviously continue current therapy. Occasionally patients are digitalized intra-operatively particularly if an extensive tumour necessitates resection within the pericardium.

## References

American College of Cardiology/American Heart Association (1996) Guidelines for perioperative evaluation for noncardiac surgery. *Circulation;* **93:** 1278–1317.

Baier H. (1980) Assessment of unilateral lung function. *Anesthesiology;* **52:** 240–247.

Crapo R.O. (1994) Pulmonary–function testing. Current concepts. *N Engl J Med;* **331:** 25–30.

Goldman L. (1995) Cardiac risk in noncardiac surgery: an update. *Anesth Analg;* **80:** 810–820 (see also erratum p. 1253).

Goldman L., Caldera D.L., Nussbaum S.R. *et al.* (1977) Multifactorial index of cardiac risk in noncardiac surgical procedures. *N Engl J Med;* **297:** 845–850.

Mangano D.T. (1990) Perioperative cardiac morbidity. *Anesthesiology;* **72:** 153–184.

Nunn J.F., Milledge J.S., Chen D. and Dore C. (1988) Respiratory criteria of fitness for surgery and anaesthesia. *Anaesthesia;* **43:** 543–551.

Thomas S.D., Berry P.D. and Russell G.N. (1995) Is this patient fit for thoracotomy and resection of lung tissue? *Postgrad Med J;* **71:** 331–335.

# Chapter 7

# Anaesthesia for thoracic surgery

## Anaesthetic techniques

Anaesthetic techniques for thoracic surgery (Table 7.1) are little different from those employed for other forms of major surgery. Anaesthesia is induced intravenously and the choice of agent is not critical for long procedures involving lung resection. Endobronchial intubation is performed following the administration of a non-depolarizing muscle relaxant such as pancuronium for lung resection or a shorter acting drug for less major procedures such as videoscopic surgery. There is still an indication to use the depolarizing agent suxamethonium, however, if a difficult laryngeal intubation is considered likely or if another airway problem such as bronchopleural fistula is apparent.

Maintenance of anaesthesia is usually with an inhalational agent such as isoflurane, combined with an intravenous opioid where appropriate. If epidural opioids are to be used to provide postoperative pain relief then it is preferable to avoid the use of intravenous opioids during surgery. The subject of postoperative analgesia, and its impact on intra-operative management, is discussed fully in Chapter 9.

Controversy remains surrounding the choice between inhalational anaesthesia and intravenous techniques for use during one-lung ventilation. In practice there is little difference in the oxygenation achieved with either technique, but this subject is discussed in more detail in the section on one-lung anaesthesia (see below).

## Monitoring

Monitoring and vascular access for major thoracic surgery should be comprehensive, as listed in Table 7.2. Pulmonary artery catheters can only be placed in the lung contralateral to surgery if radiological screening facilities are readily available. This is not considered justifiable or necessary in routine clinical practice.

**Table 7.1 Anaesthetic techniques suitable for lung resection**

*Induction*
  Propofol
    Satisfactory in most patients; repeat as necessary to prevent awareness during pre-operative
    bronchoscopy.
    Target controlled infusion (TCI) useful for longer procedures
  Etomidate
    Consider its use in the elderly or those with cardiovascular instability

*Neuromuscular blockade*
  Choice of non-depolarizing agent not critical
  Pancuronium, rocuronium, vecuronium and atracurium all suitable agents
  Histamine release with atracurium not usually a problem, but advisable to avoid in asthmatics
  Consider suxamethonium for difficult intubation or airway fistula

*Maintenance of anaesthesia*
  Inhalational agent
    Isoflurane most suitable (avoid halothane)
  Inspired gas mixture – 50% oxygen in nitrous oxide or air
    Avoid nitrous oxide with abnormal air spaces
    Increase inspired oxygen concentration for OLV
  Total intravenous anaesthesia (TIVA)
    Propofol by target controlled infusion (TCI)

*Intra-operative analgesia*
  Intravenous opiates
    Morphine (0.1–0.2 mg/kg) based on age/physical status, etc. – supplement at end of surgery
    Fentanyl (5–15 µg/kg) – alternative
    Avoid intravenous opioids if epidural opioids used
  Epidural analgesia
    Thoracic/high lumbar/lumbar – all feasible
    Opioids alone or combined with low-dose local anaesthetic agent most popular (see Chapter 9)

**Table 7.2 Monitoring – major thoracic surgery**

Electrocardiogram (ECG)

Pulse oximetry

End-tidal gas analysis
  Oxygen
  Carbon dioxide (invaluable during OLV)
  Inhalational agent

Flow/volume loop
  Useful, if available, especially during OLV
  Display of ventilator pressures and volumes a satisfactory substitute

Invasive arterial pressure measurement
  Arterial cannula in radial artery contralateral to side of surgery most practical because of
  position of the arm

Invasive central venous pressure measurement/volume line
  Quadruple lumen catheter in the internal jugular vein on the side of surgery preferable

Nasopharyngeal temperature
  Heat loss significant during thoracotomy
  Warming mattresses not efficient with patient in lateral position
  Warm-air heating devices preferable

Urinary output measurement
  Urinary catheter appropriate for long procedures
  Consider also if epidural analgesia is to be used or if renal function is poor

## Posture – the lateral thoracotomy position

Thoracotomy for lung resection is usually carried out with the patient in a lateral position. The patient remains supine, until endobronchial intubation and the insertion of arterial and central venous lines is complete, and is then turned into the lateral position after the side of surgery has been confirmed. The lower shoulder is pulled through anteriorly, allowing the flexed lower arm to be tucked under the pillow supporting the head. The upper arm is extended and placed over the head to pull the scapula away from the site of operation without stretching the brachial plexus (Fig. 7.1). Some surgeons, particularly those using a more anterior muscle-sparing incision, prefer to place the upper arm in a raised arm support attached to the head end of the operating table.

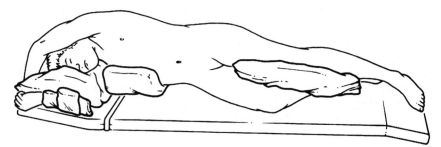

**Fig. 7.1** The lateral thoracotomy position. Reproduced with permission from Aitkenhead A.R. and Jones R.M. (eds) *Clinical Anaesthesia* (1996) Churchill Livingstone

Stability of the pelvis is achieved by flexing the lower leg at the hip and knee while the upper leg, padded by a pillow, is kept relatively straight. Further stability can be achieved with chest and pelvic supports and a wide strap provides additional support if placed across the pelvis and anchored on both sides of the operating table. Alternatively, the patient can be stabilized on a mattress which conforms to body contours and becomes rigid once its air has been evacuated. We mainly rely on a mattress at chest level which, once it has been evacuated, prevents gross movement of the thorax in the lateral position.

## Endobronchial intubation

It is accepted UK practice to place a double lumen endobronchial tube in the lung contralateral to surgery in order to facilitate lung resection. Indications for endobronchial intubation theoretically range from absolute to relative (Table 7.3) but in practice the majority of surgeons expect the provision of one-lung anaesthesia to facilitate surgery. The advent of video-assisted thoracoscopic surgery (VATS) has increased the use of endobronchial intubation because it is mandatory to collapse the lung on the side of thoracoscopic surgery in order to allow safe access via telescope and instrumentation ports (see also Chapter 8).

Bronchial blockers were used historically as an alternative to the use of double lumen or even single lumen endobronchial tubes. We occasionally use a Fogarty embolectomy catheter as a bronchial blocker in children. In adults, a bronchial blocker combined with an endotracheal tube (Univent tube) has gained some popularity and this is discussed below.

**Table 7.3 Indications for endobronchial intubation**

| | |
|---|---|
| Absolute | Fistula or rupture of major airways |
| | Lung transplantation |
| | Video-assisted thoracoscopic surgery (VATS) |
| | Massive intra-pulmonary bleeding |
| | Profuse secretions |
| | Lung cysts |
| | Lung resection |
| | Thoracic aortic/spinal surgery |
| | Oesophageal surgery |
| Relative | Open pleurectomy |

Indications range from absolute to relative. In practice one-lung ventilation is used to facilitate the majority of the above procedures if satisfactory oxygenation can be maintained

## Double lumen endobronchial tubes

Double lumen endobronchial tubes are derived from the original Carlens tube which was introduced in 1949 to allow measurement of lung volumes separately in the two lungs (differential bronchospirometry). The tube was later used intra-operatively to facilitate thoracic surgery.

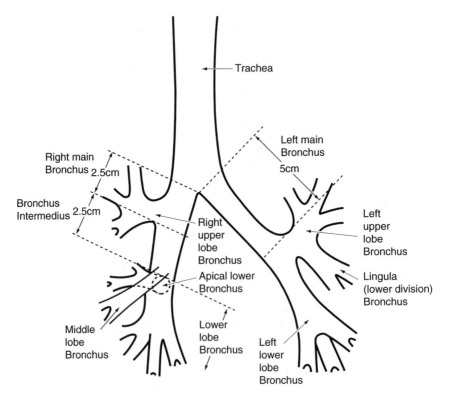

**Fig. 7.2** Anatomy of the tracheobronchial tree

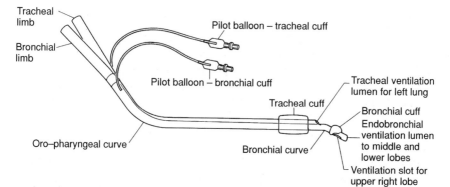

**Fig. 7.3** Basic pattern of a right-sided double-lumen endobronchial tube. Reproduced with permission from Gothard J.W.W. (1993) *Anaesthesia for Thoracic Surgery,* 2nd edn. Blackwell Scientific Publications

**Table 7.4 Comparison of Robertshaw and Bronchocath endobronchial tubes**

| *Robertshaw (Phoenix Medical Ltd)* | *Bronchocath (Mallinckrodt)* |
| --- | --- |
| *Construction*<br>Red rubber re-usable or disposable (coated) rubber<br><br>Bronchial limb and cuff colour-coded blue | *Construction*<br>Plastic disposable<br><br>Low-pressure/high-volume cuffs<br><br>Colour-coded blue bronchial cuff and bronchial limb |
| *Sizes*<br>Right and left<br>Large, medium, small, extra-small | *Sizes*<br>Right and left<br><br>35-, 37-, 39- and 41-French gauge<br><br>Left 28-French gauge |
| *Features*<br>'Bite-block' where tracheal and bronchial limbs fuse are designed to sit at level of teeth – in practice this may be too deep<br><br>Slot in bronchial cuff (21 mm) almost twice the length of Bronchocath tubes, therefore more likely to be opposite the right upper lobe orifice | *Features*<br>Depth of insertion variable<br>Length markers on side of tube<br><br>Right upper lobe ventilation slot is only 11 mm in 41-French gauge tube<br><br>Easier to use with FOB. Standard anaesthetic FOB will pass down 35-French gauge tube |
| *Clinical use*<br>These large bulky tubes are easy to insert and much less likely to move intra-operatively than plastic tubes<br><br>They are not as easy to manipulate with a FOB, and a small anaesthetic FOB (tip size 3.8 mm) will not pass down the smaller sizes of tube<br><br>Smaller anaesthetic bronchoscopes are planned by the manufacturers | *Clinical use*<br>Not as stable after insertion as Robertshaw tubes. Broader size range useful, especially in women<br><br>Malleable plastic tube also useful for 'rail-roading' techniques with FOB and difficult laryngeal intubation |

The majority of tubes are now available in right and left forms and are based on a later, more practical, design by the British anaesthetist Robertshaw (1965). The tubes incorporate an endobronchial limb, a tracheal limb and both tracheal and bronchial cuffs. They are shaped to fit into the airway with a proximal oropharyngeal curve and a distal bronchial curve. The bronchial cuff design is different between left and right tubes because the right upper lobe orifice comes off much sooner after the carina in the right main bronchus than the left upper lobe orifice in the left main bronchus (Fig. 7.2). Most right tubes have a ventilation slot (or similar arrangement) built into, or distal to, the right bronchial cuff in order to facilitate right upper lobe ventilation. Left tubes do not have this feature because of the longer left main bronchus. The basic pattern of a right double lumen endobronchial tube is shown in Fig. 7.3.

Endobronchial tubes are made to a similar pattern by numerous different manufacturers. There are significant design differences between makes, however, and Table 7.4 lists the features of two types of endobronchial tube (Robertshaw and Bronchocath) commonly used in the UK. Table 7.5 illustrates differences between different types of left endobronchial tube and Table 7.6 summarizes our current preferences for different endobronchial tubes in various clinical circumstances. In practice it is useful to use two different types of tube and become familiar with their features. The tube can then be matched to different

**Table 7.5 Left-sided double lumen endobronchial tubes: dimensions of the left endobronchial segment**

| Make | Size (French gauge) | Measured length (mm) | Actual length (mm) |
|------|------|------|------|
| Rusch | 41 FG | 24 | 23 (2) |
| Bronchocath | 29 FG | 29 (3) | 27.5 (3) |
| Sheridan | 41 FG | 35 (3) | 35 (2) |
| Robertshaw (Phoenix) | Large | 56 | – |

Measurements are from the proximal end of the bronchial cuff to the tip of the tube
Variability (+/-) is shown in brackets
Comment: the Robertshaw tube has the longest left endobronchial segment and might be more likely to obstruct the left upper lobe orifice. This tube is relatively more bulky than the majority of disposable tubes, however, and therefore may not be advanced as easily into the distal left main bronchus (see also Table 7.7)
Source: Watterson and Harrison (1996)

**Table 7.6 Authors' choice of endobronchial tube – clinical practice**

Men and large women
  Large or medium Robertshaw tube

Small women
  35/37 FG Bronchocath (or similar) tube
  Small Robertshaw will not take standard anaesthetic FOB (Olympus LF-2)

'Side' of tube
  Insert contra-lateral to side of lung resection
  For other types of surgery use left-sided tube where possible

Difficult intubation/distorted bronchial anatomy
  Use malleable plastic disposable tube (e.g. Bronchocath) (facilitates use of a bougie and FOB)

**Table 7.7 Recommendations for size and length of left-sided double lumen tubes**

Length of tube

Male/females 170 cm tall: insert tube to a depth of 29 cm

For every 10 cm increase in height: increase depth of insertion 1 cm

Size of tube – from measured tracheal width

| Width of trachea (mm) | Tube size (French gauge) |
| --- | --- |
| ≥18 | 41 FG |
| ≥16 | 39 FG |
| ≥15 | 37 FG |
| ≥14 | 35 FG |

Brodsky et al., 1991, 1996
Brodsky et al. (1996) advocated the largest size of tube possible. Tracheal diameter was measured from a PA chest X-ray. This requires correction for the projection and distance of the patient from the X-ray plate, etc.
The above lengths and sizes are not necessarily applicable to right-sided tubes, but may give some guidance. Fibre-optic bronchoscopy should be used to check the position of either side of tube (but especially right tubes) if there is any doubt regarding accuracy of placement

clinical circumstances. The size of tube to be used, and depth of insertion of certain makes of tube are somewhat empirical, but obviously based to some extent on the age, weight, height and sex of the patient. Guidelines for size of left-side tubes are listed in Table 7.7. The final decision regarding the size of tube may have to be made on a trial and error basis. Once the initial choice of tube is in place, its position is checked clinically and by fibre-optic bronchoscopy (see below) and this may show that a different size of tube is indicated.

## Placement of double lumen endobronchial tubes

Double lumen tubes are usually placed in the lung contralateral to surgery in the context of lung resection. Left-sided tubes are placed where possible for other types of surgery to overcome the problem of right upper lobe ventilation.

Double lumen tubes are introduced into the larynx in the normal way with the aid of a laryngoscope. The relatively rigid and curved endobronchial tube may be deflected away from the larynx by the upper incisor teeth. In these circumstances it can be helpful to use a bougie to rail-road the tube into the larynx even though the intubation would be straightforward with a standard endotracheal tube. Once in the larynx the tube is advanced 'blindly' (after removing any stilette provided) with a twisting motion towards the side of insertion. The curved endobronchial portion of the tube is usually deflected at the carina and passes into the appropriate main bronchus as the tube is advanced.

Once in place the tracheal cuff is inflated whilst both lungs are ventilated and the seal checked in the usual way. The tracheal limb of the double lumen tube is then opened to air and the double lumen catheter mount clamped so that only the bronchial limb is ventilated. The bronchial cuff is then inflated with a minimum amount of air to seal the cuff and eliminate any leak of gas from the intubated lung up through the open tracheal limb. This step is important for two reasons. Firstly, a good seal is required to establish satisfactory one-lung anaesthesia during surgery and secondly bronchial rupture has been reported in relation to overinflation of the bronchial cuff, particularly with a left-sided tube.

During the above process the position of the tube is checked by observing chest movements with inflation/deflation and by alternate auscultation of both lung fields, paying particular attention to the left upper zone with a left tube and the area of the right upper lobe with a right tube. Auscultation is also carried out with first the tracheal limb, and then the endobronchial limb, occluded via the catheter mount to ascertain that isolation of the lungs has been achieved. Finally, the change in airway pressure is noted when one-lung ventilation is commenced. These checks are repeated after the patient has been turned into the lateral position for thoracotomy, because it is not uncommon for the tube to move during this manoeuvre.

There is increasing evidence that clinical checks of tube position, as described above, are inaccurate and that it is preferable to check the position of endobronchial tubes with a fibre-optic bronchoscope (FOB). Analysis of flow/volume and pressure/volume loops during two-lung and then one-lung ventilation has been described as an alternative or complementary approach to the diagnosis of tube malposition. This analysis is, perhaps, a more sophisticated and objective version of the anaesthetist's 'feel' of the reservoir bag during manual ventilation.

## Fibre-optic bronchoscopy and double lumen tube placement

The introduction of slim, relatively inexpensive, FOB/laryngoscopes such as the Olympus LF-2 has made the routine inspection of endobronchial tubes a practical possibility.

The LF-2 is robust and has a tip of 3.8 mm which can be passed down the lumen of endobronchial tubes as small as the 35-French gauge Bronchocath provided the internal plastic moulding is smooth. It will not, however, pass down a small Robertshaw tube and a paediatric FOB is required to check the position of this size of tube.

The FOB can be used to place the endobronchial tube under direct vision from the outset in patients who are difficult to intubate or when the tube cannot be located blindly in the appropriate bronchus. In the latter situation it is a relatively simple task to insert a double lumen tube into the trachea, locate the appropriate main bronchus with a FOB passed down the tube and then 'rail-road' or slide the tube into position over the bronchoscope (Fig. 7.4). The flexibility of plastic tubes is a distinct advantage when the FOB is used in this way.

In the majority of cases the FOB will be used to check the position of tubes following blind placement. The sequence for checking the position of a double lumen tube is as follows. The FOB (Fig. 7.5) is first passed down the tracheal lumen of the double lumen tube to check there is a clear view of the main bronchus of the lung to be operated upon and that the bronchial cuff is not herniating over the carina. (The bronchial cuff of the majority of tubes is coloured blue for easy endoscopic identification.) The FOB is then passed down the endobronchial limb to ensure that the upper lobe orifice is not obstructed on the left and that the ventilation slot of a right tube is apposed to the upper lobe orifice (Fig. 7.6). If any manipulation of the tube is necessary the tracheal lumen should be rechecked. It is also advisable to repeat the procedure after the patient has been positioned for surgery because the tube can move during the turning process.

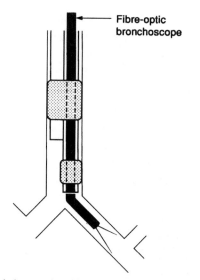

**Fig. 7.4** Positioning a double-lumen tube with the fibre-optic bronchoscope. Reproduced with permission from Aitkenhead A.R. and Jones R.M. (eds) *Clinical Anaesthesia* (1996) Churchill Livingstone

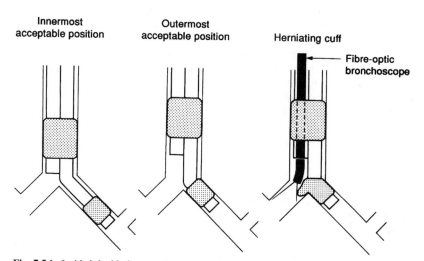

**Fig. 7.5** Left-sided double-lumen tube. Reproduced with permission from Aitkenhead A.R. and Jones R.M. (eds) *Clinical Anaesthesia* (1996) Churchill Livingstone

Despite accurate initial placement of endobronchial tubes, there is no doubt that movement can occur during surgery. This is particularly likely to occur if there is extensive surgical dissection of hilar and carinal lymph nodes for staging purposes. Rubber tubes such as the Robertshaw seem to move less than disposable plastic tubes but in general they are bulkier and less appropriate for small patients.

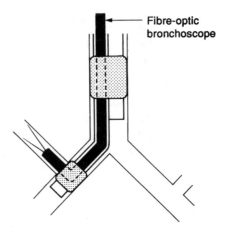

Fibre-optic
bronchoscope

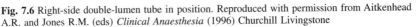

**Fig. 7.6** Right-side double-lumen tube in position. Reproduced with permission from Aitkenhead A.R. and Jones R.M. (eds) *Clinical Anaesthesia* (1996) Churchill Livingstone

If a tube is thought to have moved during surgery because of problems with one-lung ventilation or an inability to collapse the lung being operated on, repositioning can be difficult. It is useful to note the length of the tube at the teeth when it is first placed because this reference value can be used later to estimate whether the tube has slipped in or out of the main bronchus. The FOB can be used intra-operatively to recheck the position of the tube provided it does not interfere with the surgery or compromise oxygenation. It can be more difficult to identify structures at this time, however, because of the presence of blood and secretions. If the tube has slipped out of the main bronchus this can often be identified by the surgeon once the surrounding lymph nodes have been cleared. The tube can then be re-advanced into position by the anaesthetist with the surgeon guiding it, by palpation, into the appropriate bronchus.

### Univent tube (bronchial blockade)

The Univent tube comprises an endotracheal tube with a moveable bronchial blocker attached (Fig. 7.7). It was introduced into clinical practice by Inoue and co-workers in 1982.

The tube is made in a variety of sizes for use in adults. It comprises a tracheal tube with a small channel through the anterior internal wall which holds a moveable bronchial blocker with a low-pressure, high-volume cuff. The tube is placed in the trachea in the usual way and the blocker advanced, preferably under FOB control, to block the appropriate main or lobar bronchus. The blocker is then locked in place.

In the absence of commercial alternatives the Univent tube is now the standard type of bronchial blocker used in adult practice. It does have the major advantage that individual lobes can be blocked off but other perceived advantages seem more theoretical than real (Table 7.8). The Univent tube has achieved some popularity in North America but has not supplanted the use of double lumen endobronchial intubation for routine surgery in the UK.

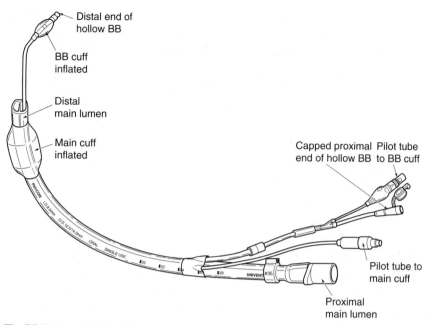

**Fig. 7.7** Univent tube – combined endotracheal tube and bronchial blocker (BB)

**Table 7.8 Univent tube – combined endotracheal tube and bronchial blocker**

| Advantages | Disadvantages |
| --- | --- |
| Lobar blockade possible | Less versatile than DLT, e.g. problem of pneumonectomy and sleeve resection |
| Ease of use for difficult intubation | |
| Facilitates aspiration of secretions | Inflation/deflation of the lung more difficult |
| Elimination of tube exchange if ventilation continued postoperatively | Blocker can migrate |
| | More expensive than DLT |

## Ventilation during thoracotomy

In the awake subject in the lateral position, blood flow to the dependent lung increases to approximately 60% of the total because of the effect of gravity on the low-pressure pulmonary vasculature. This increase in blood flow is matched by an increase in ventilation as the lower lung is on the steep part of the pressure–volume curve and the lower diaphragm, which is pushed into the chest by the abdominal contents, contracts more effectively from a position of mechanical advantage.

During anaesthesia in spontaneously breathing patients the situation changes. There is a reduction in functional residual capacity (FRC) and both lungs decrease in volume. The non-dependent upper lung now moves to the steeper part of the pressure–volume curve and receives more ventilation. Additionally, there is loss of diaphragmatic tone. The result of these changes is that the upper, non-dependent, lung is preferentially ventilated whilst the increased pulmonary blood flow to the lower lung continues.

Paralysis and intermittent positive pressure ventilation (IPPV) are used during thoracotomy to overcome the problems of the open pneumothorax created by surgery. The compliance of the non-dependent lung remains higher than that of the lower lung during IPPV so that preferential ventilation continues to the upper lung and may be further accentuated when the chest is opened.

One-lung ventilation is employed at various times during lung resection primarily to improve surgical access to the upper non-ventilated lung. This eliminates preferential ventilation but creates a far more serious problem of ventilation/perfusion mismatch.

## Physiology of one-lung anaesthesia

### Venous admixture

Pulmonary blood flow continues to the upper lung during one-lung anaesthesia, creating a true shunt in a lung where there is blood flow to the alveoli but no ventilation. This shunt is the major cause of hypoxaemia during one-lung ventilation, although the alveoli with low ventilation/perfusion ratios in the dependent lung contribute to some extent. The blood to the upper lung cannot take up oxygen and therefore retains its poorly oxygenated mixed venous composition. This mixes with oxygenated blood in the left atrium causing venous admixture and lowering arterial oxygen tension ($PaO_2$). Total venous admixture can be calculated from the shunt equation (Nunn, 1993) which estimates what proportion of the pulmonary blood flow would have bypassed ventilated alveoli to produce the arterial blood gas values for a particular patient. In published work on one-lung anaesthesia, the terms venous admixture and shunt (Qs/Qt) are used synonymously.

Venous admixture increases from a baseline value of approximately 10–15% during two-lung ventilation to a level of 30–40% during one-lung ventilation. The $PaO_2$ can be maintained in the safe range of 9–16 kPa with an inspired oxygen concentration between 50 and 100% in the majority of patients. In individual patients, however, the $PaO_2$ may fall considerably lower than this, despite a high inspired oxygen concentration. This variation is hardly surprising considering the number of interrelated physiological factors that come into play.

### Role of hypoxic pulmonary vasoconstriction

Hypoxic pulmonary vasoconstriction (HPV) is a homeostatic mechanism whereby pulmonary blood flow is diverted away from hypoxic areas of lung, thereby optimizing oxygenation of the arterial blood (Eisenkraft, 1994). The major stimulus for HPV is hypoxia both in the alveoli (low $PaO_2$) and blood perfusing the lungs (low mixed venous oxygen). The precise mechanism of HPV remains unknown but it appears to be produced by each smooth muscle cell in the wall of the pulmonary artery responding to oxygen tension in its vicinity. The smooth muscle in the wall of the arteries depolarizes and develops spontaneous electrical activity in response to hypoxia. Nitric oxide production may be inhibited by hypoxia so this also could be implicated in the mechanism of HPV.

HPV is not related to innervation of the lung as it occurs after lung transplantation. It is inhibited in a variety of pulmonary pathologies including adult respiratory distress syndrome (ARDS) and pneumonia.

Many other factors inhibit HPV. These include pulmonary vasodilator drugs, high pulmonary vascular pressure, alkalosis, acidosis, hypothermia, positive end expiratory pressure (PEEP), volatile anaesthetic agents and handling of the lung.

*In vitro* experiments have clearly shown that volatile anaesthetic agents inhibit HPV but in *in vivo* studies it has been difficult to demonstrate inhibition. This is because, although volatile agents do depress HPV directly, they also enhance HPV indirectly by reducing cardiac output. (As cardiac output drops there is an enhancement of the HPV response.) There is, therefore, an apparent unchanged HPV response in the presence of volatile anaesthetic agents during one-lung anaesthesia.

Intravenous anaesthetic agents do not inhibit HPV but the majority of studies have failed to demonstrate a significant benefit, in terms of arterial $PaO_2$, when they are used to provide anaesthesia during one-lung ventilation.

HPV seems, on current evidence, to play little role in reducing hypoxaemia during the time it takes to complete the average lung resection. It must also be remembered, when reading the literature, that handling of the lung reduces HPV and this may have a very significant effect in clinical practice. Potent inhaled anaesthetic agents such as isoflurane are not contraindicated during one-lung ventilation and may even be desirable because of their bronchodilator properties and ease of use. Significant inhibition of HPV is more likely with halothane and therefore this drug, although now rarely used in adult practice, should be avoided altogether during lung resection.

Finally, despite the comments above, there may be some cases where, if $PaO_2$ is very low during one-lung ventilation, it is worth changing from an inhalational anaesthetic to an intravenous technique. In practice this probably means substituting an isoflurane-based anaesthetic with a total intravenous anaesthesia (TIVA) technique using propofol, and monitoring its effect on arterial oxygenation.

### Cardiac output

Changes in cardiac output are likely to affect arterial oxygenation during thoracotomy. If oxygenation remains steady, a decrease in cardiac output creates a reduced mixed venous oxygen content. Some of this desaturated blood is shunted during one-lung ventilation and further exacerbates arterial hypoxaemia. Cardiac output can decrease for a number of reasons during thoracotomy. These include blood loss, fluid depletion, the use of high inflation pressures, the application of PEEP to the dependent lung and the use of PEEP to the lower lung combined with continuous positive airways pressure (CPAP) to the upper lung.

Simple measures such as replacement of blood loss, attention to fluid balance and adjustment of ventilation can help maintain cardiac output. Surgical manipulation and retraction around the mediastinum, causing a reduction in venous return, are probably the commonest causes of a sudden drop in cardiac output during lung resection. Hence the requirement for invasive arterial and venous pressure monitoring.

### Pre-operative lung function

Diseased lung may have a considerably reduced blood supply as a result of hypoxic pulmonary vasoconstriction or, in some circumstances, for physical reasons such as collapse, consolidation, cavitation or infitration by tumour.

Patients with poor lung function are sometimes accepted for lung resection on the basis that their diseased lung is contributing little to gas exchange. If this type of pulmonary disease is largely confined to the side of surgery, one-lung anaesthesia may have little effect on gas exchange. Conversely patients with near normal lung function are more likely to be hypoxic during one-lung anaesthesia. In a classic study by Kerr et al. (1974) it was reported that patients undergoing lung resection tended to have better arterial oxygenation during one-lung anaesthesia than those undergoing non-resection procedures such as oesophageal surgery. It was presumed that in the latter group an essentially normal lung was being collapsed to provide surgical access. Katz et al. (1982) also found that patients with a pre-operative $FEV_1$ nearest the predicted normal value were more likely to be hypoxic during one-lung anaesthesia.

### Management of one-lung ventilation (OLV)

It is of paramount importance to ventilate the dependent single lung optimally during one-lung anaesthesia. In principle adequate ventilation should be established in such a way as to minimize intra-alveolar pressure and therefore prevent diversion of pulmonary blood flow to the upper, non-ventilated, lung. In practice this is not always easy to achieve.

We usually use an inspired oxygen concentration ($FIO_2$) of 50% (0.5) during thoracic surgery, with an inspired gas mixture of oxygen/nitrous oxide or air/oxygen. After OLV is established we increase the oxygen concentration to as high as 100%, if required (see below). Other authors, particularly North Americans, recommend 100% oxygen from the outset.

The majority of operating theatre ventilators are of the volume-controlled type. In order to minimize mean intra-alveolar pressure a tidal volume of approximately 8–10 ml/kg is chosen initially with a conventional inspired/expired ratio (I:E ratio) of 1:2. If the minute volume is kept the same for OLV as it was during two-lung ventilation elimination of carbon dioxide is rarely a problem. A certain amount of hypercapnia is tolerated if necessary, however, and this can be monitored by end-tidal readings.

If inflation pressure is particularly high at the onset of OLV (i.e. more than $35 \, cmH_2O$) it may be necessary to reduce the tidal volume and/or reassess the position of the double lumen tube. Hyperinflation of the lungs (volutrauma) is probably more damaging to the lungs than barotrauma and should be avoided if at all possible during OLV because of its part in the aetiology of post-pneumonectomy pulmonary oedema. There is, however, limited evidence (Tugrul et al., 1997) that pressure-controlled ventilation may be more appropriate for OLV. This method of ventilation can obviously be useful in limiting airway

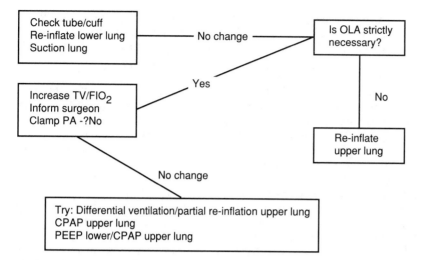

**Fig. 7.8** One-lung anaesthesia – practical management of severe hypoxia

pressures but, as previously mentioned, most operating theatre ventilators do not currently provide this facility.

If inflation pressure remains high it may be helpful to analyse a flow/volume loop or at least manually inflate the dependent lung to get 'a feel' for the compliance. A marked reduction or disappearance of the end-tidal carbon dioxide trace at this stage usually means there is a major problem with tube position or bronchial cuff inflation.

Should arterial oxygen saturation drop below 90% there are a number of steps which can be taken to improve the situation (Fig. 7.8). We initially check the position of the double lumen tube and readjust this as necessary. (When OLV becomes one-lobe ventilation hypoxaemia is inevitable.) Suction and manual re-inflation of the dependent lung may also be helpful at this stage.

The above steps may fail to improve oxygenation and therefore the inspired oxygen concentration is increased up to 100%, as necessary, taking steps to prevent patient awareness. The increase in inspired oxygen concentration cannot affect the 'true shunt' through the upper lung but will improve oxygenation via the alveoli with low ventilation/perfusion ratios in the lower lung. If this step fails to improve oxygenation it may be prudent to re-inflate the upper lung at this stage, providing the surgeon is happy to tolerate this.

In theory the shunt can be eliminated during OLV by clamping the pulmonary artery in the upper lung. This is impractical during surgery for lung cancer, however. By the time the pulmonary artery is fully dissected and exposed for clamping the period of OLV is nearly at an end. Attempts to clamp the artery earlier would be detrimental to the principles of cancer surgery, because dissection of nodes within the hilum and around the pulmonary artery needs to be carried out in a systematic manner.

Insufflation of oxygen to the upper lung via a CPAP circuit or even partial re-inflation of the upper lung with oxygen will improve oxygenation during OLV. This supplemental oxygen is taken up by the blood flow remaining to the upper lung and therefore the shunt fraction is decreased. CPAP can be applied at approximately 5–10 cmH$_2$O via commercially available CPAP circuits or, more simply, oxygen can be insufflated via a suction catheter to a partially re-inflated lung. The main drawback of this technique is that the lung becomes distended and may hinder surgery.

PEEP applied to the lower lung is not generally helpful in improving oxygenation, presumably because it tends to divert pulmonary blood flow to the upper non-ventilated lung. Some authors recommend the use of PEEP to the lower lung combined with CPAP to the upper lung to overcome this problem. In practice it is rarely necessary to use this combination of techniques during the course of a lung resection of average duration. This technique may improve arterial oxygenation but the PEEP/CPAP combination is likely to decrease cardiac output and reduce oxygen delivery.

As stated above, PEEP is statistically unlikely to improve oxygenation during OLV in the majority of patients. A recent study, however, (Cohen and Eisenkraft, 1996), albeit in a small number of patients, suggested that PEEP may be beneficial in those patients with a PaO$_2$ in the lower range (below 80 mmHg or 10.6 kPa). The authors theorize that if PEEP restores FRC to normal from an initially low level in hypoxic patients the pulmonary vascular resistance should decrease. This results in increased blood flow through the ventilated lung, a decreased shunt and an improvement in arterial oxygenation. Lower lung PEEP may therefore be useful in these circumstances and should not be dismissed as a possible therapeutic option. However, if PEEP increases the FRC from an initially normal value, pulmonary vascular resistance would increase and a larger proportion of the blood flow would be shunted through the non-dependent lung, resulting in a decrease in PaO$_2$.

In the face of persistent arterial hypoxaemia during OLV it may be pertinent to ask, 'What is a low PaO$_2$ for this patient?' We take a figure of 90% oxygen saturation below which we start worrying about the effects of hypoxia on cerebral, cardiac and renal function and general tissue oxygenation. This is an arbitrary figure, however, which is affected by a variety of factors, including acidosis and temperature. In addition, many patients will have a low PaO$_2$ when measured breathing air pre-operatively, hence the usefulness of this pre-operative measurement.

Arterial hypoxaemia is obviously undesirable but in the anaesthetized patient it may be preferable to accept a PaO$_2$ slightly lower than the pre-operative value, rather than undertake measures such as upper lung inflation which may hinder and prolong surgery.

### Acute lung injury and one-lung anaesthesia

Lung injury has been recognized as a potential complication of lung resection for many years and has been termed post-pneumonectomy pulmonary oedema (PPE). In its extreme form, PPE represents one cause of the acute respiratory distress syndrome (ARDS), although many patients not meeting the diagnostic criteria for ARDS fulfil those for the less severe acute lung injury (ALI) (see Table 7.9). Despite the terminology, PPE is not confined to pneumonectomy patients but also occurs following lobectomy. PPE complicates 4–7% of pneumonectomies and 1–7% of lobectomies, with a very high associated mortality of 50–100%. These statistics do not take into account the incidence of

**Table 7.9 Definitions of acute lung injury (ALI) and acute respiratory distress syndrome (ARDS)**

Acute lung injury (ALI) in post-thoracotomy respiratory failure requires the following for a diagnosis:
 An arterial oxygen tension ($PaO_2$, kPa) to inspired oxygen concentration ($FIO_2$) ratio of <40
 Diffuse, bilateral pulmonary infiltrates on chest X-ray
 A pulmonary capillary occlusion pressure (PAOP) of <18 mmHg

Acute respiratory distress syndrome (ARDS) requires the following for diagnosis:
 $PaO_2$ to $FIO_2$ ratio of <25
 Bilateral diffuse pulmonary infiltrates
 PAOP <18 mmHg

From Bernard *et al.* (1994)

**Table 7.10 Lung injury following lung resection – a retrospective study**

|  | *No. cases* | *ARDS (n = 17)* | *ALI (n = 7)* |
|---|---|---|---|
| Pneumonectomy | 103 | 5 (4.8%) | 2 (1.9%) |
| Lobectomy | 231 | 12 (5.2%) | 5 (2.2%) |
| Wedge resection | 135 | 0 | 0 |
| Total no. cases | 469 | 17 (3.6%) | 7 (1.5%) |
| Total no. deaths (overall) | – | 15 | 2 |
| % Deaths of total | – | 3.4 | 0.5 |

Summary: lung injury (ALI + ARDS) occurred in 5.1% of patients; mortality for ARDS (once established) was 88%; mortality for ALI was 29%

All cases of ALI/ARDS identified using criteria outlined in Table 7.8
Royal Brompton Hospital 1991–1994. Data courtesy of Prof T. Evans and Dr E. Williams, Dept of Critical Care, Royal Brompton Hospital, London, UK

ALI following lung resection, however. Figures for ARDS and ALI following lung resection in our own institution are summarized in Table 7.10.

The many factors which contribute to PPE are discussed further in Chapter 9. It is becoming increasingly evident, however, that ischaemia–reperfusion injury mediated by reactive oxygen species is implicated in the aetiology of pulmonary injury following lung resection (Williams *et al.*, 1996).

During OLV relative ischaemia of the non-dependent lung being operated upon is followed by re-expansion and reperfusion of the remaining lung tissue after lobectomy and by hyperperfusion of the ventilated lung after pneumonectomy. It is therefore likely that all patients undergoing lung resection and OLV are subjected to conditions under which there is an increased risk of developing lung injury. Factors that determine the degree of endothelial damage in ALI and the release of vasoactive substances such as nitric oxide (NO), and their influence in modulating HPV have yet to be elucidated. Whether further work in this field can lead to management strategies which will decrease the incidence of ALI following lung resection is also open to question.

### Newer therapeutic modalities and one-lung anaesthesia

Ventilation, as described above, is the main area in which changes are made in order to reduce hypoxia during OLV. Increasing interest is being shown in the pharmacological manipulation of pulmonary blood flow during OLV but this is at an early stage of investigation.

The pulmonary vasodilator prostaglandin $E_1$ has been selectively infused into the pulmonary artery of the ventilated lung in adult patients undergoing OLV (Chen *et al.*, 1996). This has been found to reduce venous admixture/shunt fraction (Qs/Qt), improve arterial oxygenation and lower pulmonary vascular resistance.

Selective infusion into one single pulmonary artery is relatively difficult to achieve and other workers have studied the effects of inhaled nitric oxide (NO) into the dependent, ventilated, lung during OLV. One of the first studies of this type (Wilson *et al.*, 1997) failed to show any benefit from this technique in adult patients. There is, however, some animal evidence that NO may be helpful during one-lung anaesthesia and further clinical studies are required in this area.

The NO synthase inhibitor nitro-L-arginine methyl ester (L-NAME) has been used intravenously and in nebulized form in animal experiments to block the production of NO and decrease blood flow to hypoxic areas of lung. This approach could, potentially, be used to reduce blood flow to the non-ventilated lung during one-lung anaesthesia. Again, this form of treatment is at a very early stage of investigation.

### High-frequency jet ventilation

High-frequency jet ventilation (HFJV) can be used to provide satisfactory gas exchange during thoracotomy either via an endotracheal tube or some form of endobronchial tube. HFJV provides satisfactory ventilation by either route and has the advantage of low peak airway pressures, albeit with the production of obligatory PEEP by the majority of systems. Some clinicians advocate the use of HFJV during thoracic surgery and use it on a routine basis. This method of ventilation has not been adopted widely, however. Reasons for this include difficulty with surgical access as the lung is distended and the inability to administer gaseous anaesthetic agents.

HFJV may have a role to play in the management of specific conditions and it has been advocated for a variety of procedures including bilateral bullectomy, management of bronchopleural fistula, sleeve resection of the right upper lobe and airway surgery.

## Termination of surgery and anaesthesia

### Testing of bronchial suture lines

On completion of lung resection bronchial suture lines and lung surfaces are tested for an air leak. Sterile water is instilled into the pleural cavity, following cancer surgery, to cover the bronchial suture lines. After lobectomy the remaining lobe or lobes are then suctioned prior to re-inflation. In the case of pneumonectomy very gentle suction is applied with a soft catheter to the bronchial stump. At this stage it may also be helpful to deflate the bronchial cuff. The bronchial stump is then tested for a leak as a positive pressure of approximately 30 cmH$_2$O is applied manually in a sustained manner via the ventilation circuit to both lumina of the double lumen tube (we now keep this testing pressure down for fear of increasing the risk of ALI in the postoperative period).

In the unlikely event of a leak being present gas bubbles will be seen appearing below the water level in the pleural cavity, indicating the need for further surgery.

We tend to test for lung surface leaks at a lower inflation pressure of approximately 20 cmH$_2$O. A degree of lung leak may be tolerated from a raw surface, if it is thought the remaining lung tissue will expand satisfactorily to fill the thoracic cavity, but a large leak may warrant further suturing.

### Termination of anaesthesia

After completion of lung resection and closure of the chest wall, anaesthesia is lightened and spontaneous ventilation re-established in the usual manner. Before removal of the endobronchial tube the patient is placed in a supine position.

Following lobectomy tracheo-bronchial suction is carried out, to clear secretions and blood in the bronchi of the intact lung and the remaining lobes of the operated lung. The lungs are then manually re-inflated again, also at a low pressure, with the chest drains open to an underwater seal drain. The endobronchial tube is removed when the patient's respiratory effort is satisfactory.

A similar sequence is followed after pneumonectomy but the remaining lung is re-inflated until the trachea is approximately central or slightly towards the side of surgery. The chest drain, if one has been inserted, is then clamped. If a chest drain has not been used after pneumonectomy it may be necessary to aspirate air from the hemithorax on the side of surgery in order to optimize the position of the mediastinum as judged clinically and on an early postoperative chest X-ray.

Patients are placed in the sitting position after removal of the double lumen tube and allowed to breathe oxygen-enriched air. Further postoperative care is supervised in a high-dependency area or intensive care unit.

On occasions patients may a require a period of postoperative ventilation following lung resection. If this is likely to be over a short period, for example whilst the effects of epidural or intravenous opiates are allowed to wear off, we ventilate via the double lumen tube with the bronchial cuff deflated. For a more prolonged period of ventilation, for example after a long and difficult lung resection combined with chest wall resection, we change the endobronchial tube to an endotracheal tube and ventilate conventionally keeping inflation pressures low.

# References

Bernard G.R., Artigas A., Brigham K.L. *et al.* (1994) The American–European Consensus Conference on ARDS. *Am J Respir Crit Care Med;* **149**: 818–824.

Brodsky J.B., Benumof J.L, Ehrenwerth J. and Ozaki G.T (1991) Depth of placement of left double lumen endobronchial tubes. *Anesth Analg;* **73**: 570–572.

Brodsky J.B., Macario A. and Mark B.D. (1996) Tracheal diameter predicts double lumen tube size: a method for selecting left double lumen tubes. *Anesth Analg;* **82**: 861–864.

Chen T.-L., Lee Y.-T., Wang M.-J. *et al.* (1996) Endothelin-1 concentrations and optimization of arterial oxygenation and venous admixture by selective pulmonary artery infusion of prostaglandin E$_1$ during thoracotomy. *Anaesthesia;* **51:** 422–426.

Cohen E. and Eisenkraft J.B. (1996) Positive end-expiratory pressure during one-lung ventilation improves oxygenation in patients with low arterial oxygen tensions. *J Cardiothorac Vasc Anesth;* **10:** 578–582.

Eisenkraft J.B. (1994) Anaesthesia and hypoxic pulmonary vasoconstriction. In *Recent Advances in Anaesthesia and Analgesia* (Eds Atkinson R.S. and Adams A.P.). Churchill Livingstone, Edinburgh, Vol. 18, Chapter 7, pp. 103–122.

Inoue H., Shotsu A., Ogawa J. *et al.* (1982) New device for one-lung anaesthesia: endotracheal tube with movable blocker. *J Thorac Cardiovasc Surg;* **83:** 940–941.

Katz J.A., Laverne R.G., Fairley H.B. *et al.* (1982) Pulmonary oxygen exchange during endobronchial anesthesia. *Anesthesiology;* **56:** 164–171.

Kerr J.H., Crampton Smith A., Prys-Roberts C. *et al.* (1974) Observations during endobronchial anaesthesia II: oxygenation. *Br J Anaesth;* **46:** 86–92.

Nunn J.F. (1993) *Applied Respiratory Physiology* (4th Edition). Butterworth Heinemann, London.

Robertshaw F.L. (1962) Low resistance double lumen endobronchial tubes. *Br J Anaesth;* **34:** 576–579.

Tugrul M., Camci E., Karadeniz H. *et al.* (1997) Comparison of volume controlled with pressure controlled ventilation during one-lung anaesthesia. *Br J Anaesth;* **79:** 306–310.

Watterson L.M. and Harrison G.A. (1996) A comparison of the endobronchial segment of modern left-sided double lumen tubes in anesthesia for bilateral sequential lung transplantation. *J Cardiothorac Vasc Anesth;* **10:** 583–585.

Williams E. A., Evans T.W. and Goldstraw P. (1996) Acute lung injury following lung resection: is one lung anaesthesia to blame? Editorial. *Thorax;* **51:** 114–116.

Wilson W.C., Kapelanski D.P., Benumof J.L. *et al.* (1997) Inhaled nitric oxide (40 ppm) during one-lung ventilation, in the lateral decubitus position does not decrease pulmonary vascular resistance or improve oxygenation in normal patients. (Ed. Pearl R.G.). *J Cardiothorac Vasc Anesth;* **11:** 172–176.

# Further reading

Benumof J.L. (1995) *Anesthesia for Thoracic Surgery* (2nd Edition). W. B. Saunders, Philadelphia.

Gothard J.W.W. (1993) *Anaesthesia for Thoracic Surgery* (2nd Edition). Blackwell Scientific Publications, Oxford.

Kavanagh B.P. and Sandler A.N. (1996) Anaesthesia for thoracic surgery. In *The Lung in Anaesthesia and Intensive Care* (Ed. Pearl R.G). *Clin Anaesthesiol;* **10:** 99–122. Baillière Tindall, London.

# Chapter 8

# Intra-operative management of specific thoracic procedures

## Bronchoscopy

### Indications

Isolated rigid bronchoscopy has largely been superseded by flexible fibre-optic bronchoscopy for the initial diagnosis of lung and airway disease. Fibre-optic bronchoscopy is usually carried out by respiratory physicians under local anaesthesia but rigid bronchoscopy remains the procedure of choice for surgical assessment of the airway before staging procedures such as mediastinotomy or prior to lung resection. The rigid bronchoscope is also the preferred instrument for therapeutic procedures such as removal of foreign bodies, stent insertion and resection of airway tumour. Anaesthesia for bronchoscopy and other telescopic procedures within the thorax has been the subject of a recent review (Plummer *et al.*, 1998). Our current practice is summarized below.

### Patient characteristics

Mainly patients with lung cancer presenting for lung resection or a diagnostic procedure but all patients undergoing thoracotomy, for whatever reason, are bronchoscoped prior to surgery. Patients with lung cancer are often elderly smokers and their pre-operative evaluation has been dealt with in previous chapters. Patients may also present primarily with airway pathology and they will undergo rigid bronchoscopy as an isolated procedure unless this is combined with a therapeutic procedure such as dilatation of the trachea, resection of tumour or stent insertion.

### Risk factors and pre-operative assessment

For isolated bronchoscopy and therapeutic procedures it is important to evaluate the upper airway and assess whether there is any clinical evidence of obstruction. Examination of the patient may reveal whether this obstruction is severe, for example if there is breathlessness at rest, audible stridor or use of the accessory muscles of respiration. The following investigations may also be useful in defining the degree of obstruction prior to anaesthesia:

- Lung function tests (particularly the flow/volume loop)
- Chest X-ray – with additional lateral view of the trachea
- CT or MRI scan showing main airways.

Rigid bronchoscopy may entail a degree of neck extension which is particularly hazardous in the anaesthetized and paralysed patient. A lateral neck X-ray should be checked for abnormalities in patients with rheumatoid arthritis or a history of neck problems. These X-rays can be difficult to interpret, however, and if in doubt the opinion of an experienced radiologist should be sought.

## Monitoring/vascular access

- Peripheral venous access
- ECG
- Pulse oximetry
- Non-invasive BP measurement.

Direct measurement of intra-arterial blood pressure is indicated in patients with severe upper airway obstruction and an arterial cannula should be placed percutaneously under local anaesthesia before induction of general anaesthesia. Direct arterial monitoring is also useful, and justified, for longer airway procedures such as stent insertion or resection of tumour.

## Positioning

Rigid bronchoscopy is carried out with the patient in a supine position, preferably on an easily adjustable operating table. Eyes should be protected and any vulnerable teeth or bridgework noted. The head is initially placed in a neutral position with one soft pillow in place. As the bronchoscope is advanced it may be necessary to extend the neck and this can be done by carefully moving the head-end of the operating table down. This will not be possible if there is any question of an unstable cervical spine.

## Airway and ventilatory management

The rigid bronchoscope is placed through the vocal cords by the surgeon, under direct vision. This provides a direct route for ventilation, but obviously this airway has to be 'shared' between surgeon and anaesthetist throughout the whole procedure. Main methods of providing gas exchange during rigid bronchoscopy are given below:

### Venturi injector

A high-pressure source of oxygen is intermittently injected through a fine needle at the proximal end of the bronchoscope thereby creating a Venturi effect. Air is entrained and positive pressure is produced at the distal end of the bronchoscope. Intermittent inflation/deflation provides satisfactory oxygenation and carbon dioxide clearance. The injector is usually controlled manually, although automatic control devices have been described. It is essential, if Venturi devices are used, to ensure there is an adequate opening at the proximal end of the bronchoscope to allow entrainment of air and *(most importantly, if barotrauma is to be avoided)* egress of gas during expiration. It is also important to match the injector needle size to the type of bronchoscope and oxygen pressure used (Table 8.1). This mode of ventilation is usually used in adults but some European

**Table 8.1 Maximum inflation pressure achieved with various Venturi injector systems**

| Negus bronchoscope | Injector needle (SWG) | Maximum pressure (cmH$_2$O) |
|---|---|---|
| Adult | 14 | 50 |
| Adult | 16 | 25–30 |
| Child | 19 | 14–18 |
| Suckling | 19 | 15 |

Adult Negus is equivalent to Adult Storz bronchoscope. Manual ventilation via a T-piece is preferred with paediatric Storz bronchoscopes (see text).
Oxygen driving pressure 410 kPa

centres use high frequency jet ventilation (HFJV) or a ventilating-type of bronchoscope even in adults.

## Ventilating bronchoscope

A glass slide device at the proximal end of the rigid bronchoscope allows manual positive pressure ventilation with a suitable gas mixture via a side port built into the bronchoscope (Storz type). A rubber diaphragm can replace the glass window as required so that a telescope can be used down the bronchoscope whilst ventilation is continued. This technique is ideal for use in infants and children. A T-piece circuit is attached to the side port of the bronchoscope and anaesthesia is maintained with non-cumulative gaseous agents with minimal risk of barotrauma.

## Anaesthetic technique

Anaesthesia for rigid bronchoscopy should provide the following conditions: unconsciousness, muscular relaxation, abolition of respiratory tract reflexes, ventilation and a rapid recovery. A suitable anaesthetic technique for a short isolated bronchoscopy comprises of:

● Light benzodiazepine pre-medication (omit with airway obstruction)
● Anti-sialogogue – usually not required with pre-medication (use IV glyco-pyrrolate as necessary intra-operatively)
● Intravenous induction (propofol)
● Short-acting muscle relaxant (mivacurium or suxamethonium)
● Inhalational induction preferable in children and with upper airway obstruction.

Some anaesthetists elect to spray the vocal cords with plain lignocaine (maximum of 4 ml of 4%) prior to instrumentation in an effort to minimize postoperative laryngospasm. This has only been shown to be beneficial following very short procedures.

Maintenance of anaesthesia is usually with intermittent bolus doses of an intravenous agent and in this respect propofol is an ideal drug, provided systemic blood pressure is maintained. The sympatho-adrenal response resulting from instrumentation of the upper respiratory tract during bronchoscopy is similar to that following laryngoscopy and intubation, but may be more marked, with an

**Table 8.2 Induction and maintenance of propofol anaesthesia**

*Induction*
  Propofol 1 mg/kg

*Maintenance*
  Propofol
    10 mg/kg/h for 10 minutes
    8 mg/kg/h for 8 minutes
    6 mg/kg/h continuously thereafter

Note: preferable to use target controlled infusion of propofol (TCI propofol)

increase in heart rate and both systemic and pulmonary hypertension. A study by Hill *et al.* (1991) suggested that the incidence of myocardial ischaemia may be as high as 10–15% during bronchoscopy. The same authors found that anaesthesia with propofol alone, following pethidine and atropine premedication, provided adequate haemodynamic stability during bronchoscopy and the addition of alfentanil was superfluous.

If bronchoscopy is prolonged or is to be followed by a surgical procedure a longer acting muscle relaxant such as vecuronium or atracurium can be administered. Anaesthesia is then maintained with an infusion of propofol either on the basis of a regime such as that shown in Table 8.2 or, preferably, by a target controlled infusion (TCI) technique.

### Postoperative management/complications

Muscular relaxation is reversed where necessary and the patient allowed to awaken. Oxygen is administered by face mask and the patient is nursed in the lateral position with the suppurative side down if secretions are present or if blood continues to ooze from a biopsy site. If this is not the case the patient is nursed in the sitting position. Acute airway obstruction at this stage due to laryngospasm, the presence of secretions or fragments of tumour is very rare but, if it does occur, reintubation or repeat bronchoscopy may be indicated.

## Laser bronchoscopy and diathermy resection

### Indications

Surgical laser devices are used to resect tracheobronchial tumours; alternatively a simple diathermy resection instrument incorporating a telescope can be used. These devices only clear the intraluminal portion of the tumour and therefore this surgery is usually of a palliative nature to relieve airway obstruction, breathlessness and haemoptysis. Very rarely a benign polypoid tumour with a narrow base may be completely excised with these techniques.

### Patient characteristics

These procedures are often carried out in elderly debilitated patients with severe bronchial or tracheal obstruction. ASA status may be as low as the III–IV range.

## Risk factors and pre-operative assessment

The main risk factors relate to pre-existing airway obstruction (see bronchoscopy section above) and problems of intra-operative bleeding and hypoxia due to blood and tumour fragments or even inadequate control of the airway. Pre-medication should be omitted in the majority of these patients.

## Monitoring and vascular access

As for bronchoscopy.

In severely compromised patients intra-arterial pressure monitoring should be established before induction of anaesthesia.

## Airway and ventilatory management

A variety of lasers has been used for resection of endobronchial tumours including the carbon dioxide and neodymium yttrium-aluminium-garnet (NdYAG) lasers. The thermal effect of these lasers is the main basis for their efficacy but this also has significant implications for their use during general anaesthesia. There is a considerable fire hazard when lasers are used in the presence of conventional tracheal tubes, particularly in an atmosphere of high oxygen concentration. Foil wrapped, or even metal, tracheal tubes have been used to provide an airway for laser treatment but a simpler approach is to utilize a metal rigid bronchoscope for tracheal and endobronchial tumour resection.

Following induction of anaesthesia, a rigid adult bronchoscope is introduced into the airway and Venturi ventilation commenced. Alternatively, a ventilating type of bronchoscope may be used. It may be necessary to push the bronchoscope past the tumour initially in order to provide an adequate airway or occasionally large fragments of tumour require rapid removal with biopsy forceps. A fibre-optic bronchoscope can then be passed down the bronchoscope to reach the area of tumour whilst ventilation continues. An optical fibre is then introduced down the biopsy channel of the fibre-optic instrument in order to transmit the laser beam to the required site. Biopsy forceps and suction catheters can be passed down the rigid bronchoscope intermittently to remove blood and tumour debris, thus ensuring a relatively clear airway. At times it will be necessary to suspend Venturi ventilation whilst smoke particles are sucked away from the airway.

We prefer to use a diathermy resectoscope down the rigid bronchoscope to remove tumour. This is carried out in a similar manner to that described above without the use of complex laser technology.

## Anaesthetic technique

Anaesthesia for laser therapy is carried out on the principles previously described for bronchoscopy. Following pre-oxygenation anaesthesia can usually be induced intravenously and maintained with an infusion of propofol after paralysis with atracurium or vecuronium. Induction of anaesthesia is particularly hazardous in the presence of upper airway obstruction as alluded to previously.

The theoretical advantages of an inhalational induction are rarely applicable to this type of palliative surgery carried out in elderly debilitated patients, but may be considered in extreme circumstances. In this respect sevoflurane is the agent of choice. A mixture of helium in 21% oxygen can also be used to increase alveolar oxygen supply prior to surgery. Helium is less dense than nitrogen and will therefore increase turbulent flow rates through an obstructed airway if used as the carrier gas. In practice this is rarely indicated.

We usually induce anaesthesia intravenously (for this type of extreme palliative surgery) even in the presence of significant upper airway obstruction, but only if it is considered that an airway can be rapidly established via the rigid bronchoscope. This approach relies heavily on the immediate presence of a skilled and experienced bronchoscopist. After pre-oxygenation, intravenous anaesthesia is induced slowly. Intravenous suxamethonium (rather than a non-depolarizing agent) is then given to allow rapid insertion of the bronchoscope. Once an airway as been established and ventilation commenced (and this may be via a small size of bronchoscope) a longer acting muscle relaxant can be given.

### Postoperative management/complications

Postoperative management is similar to that described following bronchoscopy. Airway problems are, however, more likely following prolonged laser therapy. Continued bleeding and the presence of tumour fragments can cause or exacerbate laryngospasm so that re-intubation is more common. A postoperative chest X-ray should be obtained to check that both lung fields are adequately expanded (if this can be reasonably expected in relation to the patient's pre-operative condition). The tracheobronchial tree may also be breached surgically during radical intraluminal dissection and the presence of a pneumothorax or mediastinal air is evidence of this. These problems may resolve without further treatment but further progression will require chest drainage and possibly the insertion of a tracheobronchial stent.

## Tracheobronchial stent insertion

### Indications

Tracheobronchial stents are used to improve and maintain airway patency in a variety of pathologies. These include tracheal stenosis following prolonged intubation or tracheostomy, narrowing at the site of bronchial anastomoses after sleeve resection or lung transplantation and as a further palliative measure following diathermy/laser resection of endobronchial tumour. Many different types of stent are available and these continue to proliferate, as this is an area of rapid development.

The original Montgomery T-tube is still used to treat proximal tracheal strictures and this allows ventilation through the upright limb via a tracheostomy. Bifurcating prostheses are available to stent the lower trachea and both main bronchi and simpler tubular plastic stents can be used in either site. Various types of expanding metal stents are now available which may or may not have an outer covering. Metal stents are conveniently inserted with a purposed-made introducer under radiological control.

## Anaesthetic technique and airway management

The anaesthetic considerations for the insertion of endobronchial and intra-tracheal stents are similar to those for laser bronchoscopy, with ventilation and maintenance of the airway being of most concern. The anaesthetic technique is as described above with some minor differences in approach to ventilation.

Venturi ventilation can be used during the majority of stent insertions, although some European colleagues prefer to use manual, positive pressure ventilation via a ventilating bronchoscope. In extreme circumstances partial cardiopulmonary bypass has been instituted to augment oxygenation prior to the insertion of tracheobronchial stents but this is very unusual. High-frequency jet ventilation has also been used during stent insertion.

Stents are initially placed through the larynx under direct vision and then advanced into the final position with the aid of grasping forceps placed through the rigid bronchoscope. As the stents are advanced there will be times when the airway becomes completely blocked and ventilation is impossible. Close co-operation between surgeon and anaesthetist is essential at this stage and if the stent cannot be positioned before hypoxaemia ensues it should be rapidly removed and the lungs reventilated. It may take several attempts before the stent is optimally placed in this manner. If a T-tube is being inserted or replaced it may be possible to use Venturi ventilation via the open tracheal limb of the tube once the distal limb is open. It is essential to ensure that expiration can occur whichever mode of ventilation is used, otherwise barotrauma will ensue with disastrous consequences.

## Postoperative management/complications

Once the stent is in place, anaesthesia is discontinued and the patient allowed to breathe spontaneously in a sitting position. A postoperative chest X-ray is mandatory.

Airway patency should be significantly improved following stent insertion. There may, however, be short-term problems relating to the presence of blood and secretions in addition to the trauma associated with instrumentation of the airway. Rarely, stents can move, particularly in the early postoperative period. Acute airway obstruction, which requires immediate re-operation, can result.

# Removal of foreign bodies from the airway

## Indications

All foreign bodies should be removed from the tracheobronchial tree. Small, inert, foreign bodies inhaled into the distal airway are unlikely to cause airway obstruction but eventually they will erode into the lung and set up a focus of infection. This will lead to a lung abscess which will require open thoracotomy, excision and possibly lobectomy.

Acute upper airway obstruction is the immediate hazard when foreign bodies are initially inhaled but they often pass deeper into the tracheobronchial tree. Here they impact and set up a local inflammatory reaction ultimately causing distal collapse and infection in the obstructed portion of lung.

Almost any small object can be inhaled once put in the mouth or held in the teeth. Fragments of poorly manufactured toys are a particular problem in children but organic material can prove even more troublesome because it swells after inhalation and may fragment, even before attempts are made to remove it. Peanuts are commonly inhaled by small children and these swell *in situ*, fragment and liberate an irritant oil which causes severe local inflammation.

### Patient characteristics

Foreign bodies are inhaled at any age but, most commonly, by children under the age of three. Adults also inhale foreign bodies, however, sometimes after alcoholic excess but occasionally as a completely unexpected event.

A specific history of inhalation may be available but this is often absent in children. Paroxysmal cough and wheeze are common presenting symptoms in children but dyspnoea, stridor and fever may also occur. A persistent chest infection which fails to clear after appropriate antibiotic therapy may warrant diagnostic bronchoscopy to exclude a foreign body in children. A chest X-ray (with inspiratory and expiratory films) may reveal obstructive emphysema as the foreign body acts as a ball-valve in a main bronchus. More often radiological appearances are non-specific, with atelectasis and consolidation or even no abnormality at all.

### Risk factors

The immediate risk of foreign body inhalation is upper airway obstruction. This is unusual but likely to be evident clinically. Pre-medication is omitted in this group of patients but atropine may be given to dry secretions.

### Monitoring/vascular access

As for bronchoscopy.

### Airway and ventilatory management

Venturi ventilation is satisfactory for adults, but care must be taken not to blow the foreign body deeper into the tracheobronchial tree. The ventilating bronchoscope (e.g. Storz) is more satisfactory for use in children.

### Anaesthetic technique

In adults the anaesthetic techniques described for bronchoscopy are satisfactory in the majority of cases. An inhalational induction may be indicated in the presence of upper airway obstruction but this is an extremely rare problem.

It is traditional to induce children who are presumed to have inhaled a foreign body with an inhalational induction. This has two advantages; firstly cumulative doses of intravenous induction agent do not interfere with a rapid awakening when the procedure is over and secondly the airway can be safely maintained up to the time of bronchoscopy. Some anaesthetists continue on from an inhalational induction to provide deep general anaesthesia in the spontaneously breathing patient. A bronchoscope can then be inserted without prior muscle relaxation.

We prefer to administer intravenous suxamethonium initially to allow easy, atraumatic, passage of the rigid bronchoscope through the vocal cords after an inhalational induction with sevoflurane. Ventilation is then gently commenced via a T-piece circuit connected to the ventilating bronchoscope. Anaesthesia can be maintained with either sevoflurane or isoflurane in a relatively high concentration of oxygen.

If manual ventilation is used muscular paralysis can be maintained with small incremental doses of suxamethonium, taking care to treat bradycardia with intravenous atropine. Should the procedure be particularly prolonged, and there are no problems with ventilation, a non-depolarizing agent can be given.

### Postoperative management/complications

Once the foreign body has been retrieved, anaesthesia is discontinued and any residual paralysis reversed. Once the child is fully awake spontaneous respiration can be permitted through the tube and endotracheal suction carried out prior to extubation. (It is often safer, particularly in infants, to allow the child to awaken with an endotracheal tube in place.) Laryngeal stridor is relatively common at this point, particularly after a prolonged procedure in a small child. If stridor is present after extubation intravenous dexamethasone and nebulized adrenaline may alleviate the problem. Re-intubation, using an endotracheal tube smaller than would normally be chosen, is necessary if severe stridor or signs of respiratory obstruction are present, however. In extreme circumstances a period of postoperative ventilation may be required. If this is the case intravenous dexamethasone is given to alleviate laryngeal and upper airway oedema. A prolonged period of postoperative ventilation may be required if an extensive pneumonia is established before removal of the foreign body. This latter scenario is rare.

# Mediastinoscopy and mediastinotomy – diagnostic procedures

## Indications

Mediastinoscopy (inspection of the mediastinum via a small incision above the suprasternal notch) is carried out via a rigid mediastinoscope to provide a diagnosis in patients with mediastinal lymphadenopathy, and to assess operability in patients with lung cancer. Approximately 80% of patients with non-small cell lung cancer are inoperable at presentation. If enlarged, abnormal mediastinal nodes are *not* present on CT or MRI scans then the patient is usually suitable for lung resection provided possible distant metastatic sites are clear. If enlarged nodes are identified it is impossible to differentiate on the scans between those that contain malignant disease and those that result from reactive hyperplasia or old inflammatory disease. Mediastinoscopy or mediastinotomy is undertaken in these patients to define their operability.

Anterior mediastinotomy, carried out via a small incision in the second interspace, allows exploration of tumours and lymph nodes of the anterior mediastinum which are inaccessible by mediastinoscopy. Left anterior mediastinotomy, in particular, is used to assess the lymph node drainage of left upper lobe tumours visually, and also by digital palpation.

## Patient population

The majority of patients will have lung cancer and the risk profile of this group has been discussed in detail in Chapter 6.

Other indications for mediastinoscopy/mediastinotomy include hilar lymphadenopathy (sarcoidosis or malignant lymphadenopathy) and mediastinal tumours. In this latter category patients with thymic tumours may prove a problem because of associated myasthenia gravis, although this is extremely rare. In addition, anterior mediastinal tumours can compromise the airway at the tracheal or bronchial level and cause superior vena caval (SVC) obstruction.

## Risk factors

The main risk factors relate to the pre-operative condition of the patient as discussed above. The most significant intra-operative complication of either mediastinoscopy or mediastinotomy is major bleeding, often related to inadvertent biopsy of a major vascular structure. In experienced hands this complication is rare but all patients must have an adequate route for intravenous infusion established prior to surgery.

## Monitoring/vascular access

- Peripheral venous access
- ECG
- Pulse oximetry
- Non-invasive BP measurement.

Theoretically blood pressure should be measured on the left arm because unreliable values may be recorded on the right if the innominate artery is compressed by the mediastinoscope. In practice this is rarely a problem.

## Positioning

Supine. A sand bag is placed under the patient's shoulders and the head, whilst placed in a head ring, is extended as far back as safety permits. A slight head-up tilt prevents venous engorgement in the few patients with superior vena caval obstruction.

## Airway and ventilatory management

Mediastinoscopy and mediastinotomy usually follow on from rigid bronchoscopy. After the bronchoscope is removed a standard endotracheal tube is inserted and IPPV continued throughout the procedure.

## Anaesthetic technique

Paralysis is maintained with a short-acting non-depolarizing agent such as atracurium or vecuronium. Anaesthesia is continued with a suitable inhalational agent such as isoflurane in an oxygen/nitrous oxide or oxygen/air mixture. Nitrous oxide is avoided if pneumothorax is a potential hazard. Postoperative pain is not a problem following mediastinoscopy but may be more evident following mediastinotomy, particularly if a section of costal cartilage has been excised. A small dose of fentanyl or alfentanil can provide adequate analgesia for either procedure but further opioid supplementation may be required postoperatively.

During mediastinotomy the pleura may be opened and this is drained during surgical closure. A large nasogastric tube is placed in the pleural space through the surgical incision and the lung is then expanded manually by the anaesthetist. As the muscle suture line is near completion a sustained inflation pressure is applied to the lung whilst the tube is withdrawn and the suture line completed.

### Postoperative management/complications

At the end of either mediastinoscopy or mediastinotomy muscular relaxation is reversed in the usual manner and spontaneous respiration re-established. The endotracheal tube is then removed following tracheobronchial suction and the patient returned to a recovery area breathing supplemental oxygen in a sitting position.

SVC or airway obstruction is likely to be exacerbated following anaesthesia and surgical biopsy. Patients with these problems need careful surveillance. Re-intubation and IPPV may be required pending medical or surgical treatment of the underlying pathology (see also mediastinal tumours – below).

## Surgery and the lung

### Lobectomy and pneumonectomy

Chapters 6, 7 and 9 discuss in some detail the anaesthetic and postoperative management of patients undergoing lung resection for lung cancer. These principles of management can be applied, with certain modifications, to patients undergoing lung resection for other pathology. For completeness this is outlined below, along with complications of lung resection which may require further surgical intervention (specifically bronchopleural fistula).

### Lobectomy

*Indications*

- Malignant and benign tumours
- Infection – bronchiectasis
- Tuberculosis (TB) and fungal infection.

*Patient characteristics*

If the lobectomy is for primary lung cancer the patients are likely to be elderly smokers as described in Chapter 6. Lobectomy for a benign tumour is uncommon but is likely to be carried out in a younger age group. Excision of metastases requiring lobectomy is also likely to be in a younger age group. Lobectomy for bronchiectasis is now uncommon but is indicated if the disease is severely debilitating and confined to one or two lobes. Fungal infection (aspergilloma) is a rare indication for lobectomy but may be undertaken to control life-threatening haemoptyses. These patients are usually in a very high-risk group because of their underlying lung pathology (fibrotic lung disease, immunosuppression and 'old' TB).

### Risk factors

These relate to the underlying pathology. Patients with bronchiectasis are admitted several days pre-operatively for physiotherapy, postural drainage and antibiotic therapy. This is aimed at reducing the volume of infected secretions in the lobe or lobes to be resected in order to minimize intra-operative spread and reduce the incidence of postoperative chest infection.

*Monitoring/vascular access*
*Anaesthetic technique*        } See Chapter 7
*Postoperative management*

### Positioning

Lobectomy is carried out with the patient in a lateral position and the operative side uppermost.

### Airway and ventilatory management

A double lumen endobronchial tube is placed in the non-operative lung for lobectomy. One-lung ventilation facilitates surgery but at times the surgeon may request reinflation of the upper lung whilst fissures are defined and dissected.

In bronchiectasis the remaining lobe or lobes on the operative side are unprotected from the spread of secretions if a double lumen tube is used. In addition infected secretions can seep past the endobronchial cuff into the opposite, dependent, lung. Repeated suction to both lungs limits this contamination, although with good pre-operative preparation this may not be a great problem.

The spread of secretions from lobe to lobe can be reduced by using bronchial blockade (e.g. a Fogarty embolectomy catheter or the Univent combined blocker and endotracheal tube) to block specific bronchi whilst continuing to ventilate the remaining lobes. We find the Fogarty catheter particularly useful when used as a bronchial blocker in children. The smallest double lumen endobronchial tube currently manufactured is a 28-French gauge left-sided Bronchocath. This is too big for most patients under approximately 35–40 kg and has impractically small ventilation lumina. Bronchial blockade with a small Fogarty catheter is therefore a practical way of achieving one-lung ventilation in children.

The main drawback of blocking techniques is that if they fail (e.g. by dislodgement) all protection from the spread of secretions is lost. Should ventilation suddenly become a problem during surgery when a blocker is in use it is probable that the blocker has moved from its original position. Deflation of the balloon should rapidly restore adequate ventilation if this is the case.

## Pneumonectomy

The usual indication for pneumonectomy is primary carcinoma of the lung. Anaesthesia and postoperative management for this procedure have been discussed previously.

Occasionally pneumonectomy is undertaken for other pathological processes such as infection or a 'completion pneumonectomy' may be carried out if there is recurrence of tumour after a previous lobectomy or even a second primary. If pneumonectomy is undertaken for infection it is usually because the lung has been totally destroyed by an underlying process such as radiotherapy or TB. A pleuro-pneumonectomy is therefore undertaken to contain the spread of infection. These operations carried out on debilitated patients can be difficult with significant blood loss. It is essential to isolate the remaining 'good' lung from the lung to be resected and a period of postoperative ventilation is usually required.

# Bronchopleural fistula

A bronchopleural fistula (BPF) is a direct communication between the tracheobronchial tree and the pleural cavity. Causes of BPF are listed in Table 8.3. In developed countries dehiscence of the bronchial stump following pneumonectomy is probably the commonest reason for patients to present for surgical repair of BPF. The incidence of BPF following pneumonectomy is, however, extremely low in specialized centres. Unfortunately the anaesthetic management of BPF remains a favoured examination topic!

Minor forms of post-pneumonectomy BPF can be cauterized at bronchoscopy with sodium hydroxide or, alternatively, may be sealed with a tissue glue. Large fistulas require surgical repair (resuture of the bronchial stump) via a lateral thoracotomy through the previous incision. Our rate of BPF is much less than 1% after pneumonectomy and in one surgeon's hands is currently zero. We occasionally are referred chronic fistulae for repair from other centres. This usually entails a period of treatment to sterilize the pneumonectomy space and then the fistula is closed surgically. The principles of anaesthetic management are similar to those described below for an acute BPF. The surgery is more

**Table 8.3 Causes of bronchopleural fistula**

Dehiscence of bronchial stump after lung resection surgery
    Lobectomy
    Pneumonectomy (most common: right>left)

Trauma
    Rupture of main bronchi
        Deceleration injury
        Usually occurs within 2–2.5 cm of the carina

Neoplasm

Inflammatory lesions
    e.g. tuberculosis

complicated, however, in that muscle flaps or omentum are placed in the chest to obliterate the space around the repaired fistula, thereby preventing re-infection. This may also be combined with a limited thoracoplasty.

## Patient characteristics

Patients are often post-pneumonectomy (3–15 days) and ASA status IV or V. Hospitals accepting major trauma may encounter patients with traumatic rupture of the major airways after high-speed road traffic accidents. These injuries are a form of BPF which usually require surgical repair.

## Pre-operative assessment

Symptoms relate to infected pneumonectomy space fluid flowing over to the remaining lung. This leads to malaise, low-grade fever, cough with wheeze and dyspnoea. Acute onset with a large BPF presents with severe dyspnoea and the patient coughing up large amounts of brownish, infected space fluid. Signs of circulatory failure also occur as a result of hypoxia and septicaemia, if the inhaled space contents were infected.

A chest X-ray usually confirms the diagnosis showing a loss of pneumonectomy space fluid and collapse/consolidation or increased shadowing in the remaining lung. With a smaller chronic fistula the chest X-ray may only show a slight drop in the level of the space fluid rather than complete loss of volume. Arterial blood gas analysis may demonstrate hypoxia, hypercarbia and metabolic acidosis.

## Initial treatment

The patient is generally resuscitated. Oxygen is administered and an intravenous infusion commenced. Most importantly the patient should be sat upright to prevent further spillover and a chest drain inserted on the pneumonectomized side to remove remaining fluid (N.B. no suction applied). The patient should be transported to theatre in a sitting position with the drain unclamped but with the underwaterseal bottle below the bed or trolley.

## Monitoring/vascular access

- Peripheral venous access
- Invasive arterial monitoring (under LA before induction)
- Central venous pressure (after induction)
- Pulse oximetry
- End-tidal gas analysis
- ECG
- Pulse oximetry
- Core temperature
- Urine output.

## Anaesthetic technique/airway management

Classically it has been taught that a post-pneumonectomy BPF should be isolated by means of an endobronchial tube placed in the remaining lung before IPPV is employed. A double lumen tube is therefore inserted in the remaining bronchus. (The size and type of tube appropriate for the original operation is usually satisfactory.) To secure the airway prior to the administration of a muscle relaxant, two methods were previously advocated:

1. Awake endobronchial intubation using local analgesia of the upper respiratory tract
2. Inhalational induction and intubation under deep inhalational anaesthesia.

The above techniques should be discussed at examinations, but in practice both are fraught with difficulty, particularly in these debilitated patients. We would now use the following technique to anaesthetize a patient with an acute BPF:

- Patient sitting upright with drain open
- Keep in semi-sitting position if possible
- Monitoring as detailed above
- Slow intravenous induction (etomidate)
- Intravenous suxamethonium
- Insertion of double lumen tube (preferably under direct vision with fibre-optic bronchoscope)
- Administer non-depolarizing muscle relaxant once lung isolated
- IPPV via endobronchial portion of the tube
- Place patient in the lateral position for thoracotomy.

### Postoperative management

Re-establishment of spontaneous respiration in the sitting position is ideal from the point of view of protecting the repaired bronchial stump from positive pressure ventilation. In practice respiratory failure is common after this procedure and it should be managed conventionally with IPPV via an endotracheal tube. HFJV has been advocated for the ventilatory management of BPF because of the low peak airway pressure generated. The evidence that this mode of ventilation is superior remains conflicting, however.

Mortality is likely to be high following repair of post-pneumonectomy BPF, but national figures are not available.

# Video-assisted thoracoscopic surgery (VATS)

Video-assisted thoracoscopic surgery (VATS) has become widely adopted to undertake various surgical procedures. These include pleurectomy, lung biopsy, drainage of effusions/talc pleurodesis and lung volume reduction surgery. Earlier enthusiasm to carry out lung resection with a VATS technique has waned, particularly in relation to carcinoma of the lung where accurate nodal dissection is vital.

VATS is perceived as being less invasive than open thoracotomy and can be carried out through a series of ports inserted through the chest wall. Postoperative pain is usually less of a problem than after open thoracotomy and length of hospital stay can be decreased for the procedures listed above. There remain reservations as to the place of VATS techniques in thoracic surgery. VATS pleurectomy, for example, appears to be a good operation which carries the benefits of a less invasive operation described above. It remains to be seen, however, whether long-term recurrence rates of pneumothorax are as low as those achievable following open pleurectomy.

## Anaesthetic considerations for VATS

Anaesthetic techniques for VATS are little different from those employed for lung resection. This has been the subject of a recent review by Plummer *et al.* (1998).

The operation is usually carried out with the patient in the lateral thoracotomy position, occasionally with the upper arm elevated in an arm rest.

It is essential to deflate the lung on the side of surgery before access ports and telescopes are introduced. We prefer to achieve this with a left-sided double lumen endobronchial tube in the majority of cases. It is extremely unlikely that this form of intubation will interfere with any biopsy/excision carried out with VATS.

Minor VATS procedures can be carried out without invasive arterial monitoring.

Postoperative pain is not so prominent following VATS procedures and therefore we rely mainly on intravenous opioids (fentanyl or morphine) for analgesia. This does not follow for all VATS procedures; for example pleurectomy can still be very painful and we may use epidural analgesia for this procedure. This also holds for lung volume reduction surgery (see below).

# Lung cysts, bullae

## Indications

Surgery for cystic lung disease concerns mainly the excision or obliteration of discrete emphysematous bullae. This is quite distinct from lung volume reduction surgery (LVRS – see below) which is indicated for widespread, heterogeneous, emphysematous lung changes.

Excision of large bullae is a major operation and may be carried out in conjunction with LVRS if there is widespread disease or as an isolated procedure. Less invasive intracavity drainage techniques have been developed therefore to obliterate isolated emphysematous bullae. These latter techniques are particularly useful in relieving symptoms in patients with marginal lung function.

## Risk factors

The main intra-operative problems with cysts and bullae are:

● They will enlarge with the uptake of nitrous oxide
● May preferentially ventilate with IPPV
● Could therefore expand and rupture, causing a tension pneumothorax.

## Anaesthetic principles and airway management

The management of anaesthesia is based on the principles described in more detail (below) for LVRS.

Endotracheal anaesthesia is employed for the lesser procedure of intracavity drainage, provided nitrous oxide is not used and ventilatory pressures are minimized.

HFJV has been advocated for the intra-operative management of bullectomy. Obligatory PEEP is produced by many jet ventilators, however, and pneumothorax can still result from their use. A more conventional approach, similar to that now used for LVRS, is to separate the two lungs with a double lumen tube. The lung contra-lateral to surgery can then be ventilated, using low inflation pressures and omitting nitrous oxide, as the bulla is excised. Bullous lung disease is often bilateral, however, and it is reasonable to ventilate both lungs up to the time the chest is open. The surgical team should be immediately available to open (or drain) the chest if a tension pneumothorax occurs in either lung.

Adequate postoperative analgesia is essential following bullectomy and intracavity drainage. Epidural analgesia should be considered.

## Lung volume reduction surgery

There has been a resurgence of interest in the surgical treatment of diffuse emphysema. This was initiated by Cooper and colleagues (1995) who undertook bilateral lung volume reduction surgery (LVRS) in 20 patients with severe chronic obstructive pulmonary disease. Their initial report detailed the surgical excision of 20–30% of the volume of each lung via a median sternotomy. There was no mortality in this small series and $FEV_1$ improved by 82% with a marked improvement in the level of dyspnoea, exercise tolerance and quality of life. Since Cooper's report, LVRS programmes have been started in many centres throughout the world.

### Indications

Brenner and colleagues (1996) stated, in a recent review, that patients selected for LVRS should have severe airflow obstruction predominantly as a result of an emphysematous process (not primary airways disease). The emphysematous process should be regionally heterogeneous to provide 'target areas' for surgical resection and therefore leave less diseased lung tissue remaining. These patients should also have marked thoracic hyperinflation and flattened diaphragms associated with air trapping. The authors also stated that predominant airways disease, hypercapnia and pulmonary hypertension were relative contraindications to surgery. Guidelines for patient selection for LVRS are shown in Table 8.4. Different centres will have their own guidelines based on local experience. But, note that lung function parameters are well below those considered acceptable for lung resection for carcinoma.

### Mechanisms of improvement in lung function after LVRS

Reducing lung volume in diffuse emphysema improves elastic recoil of the lung. This also improves airflow by increasing traction on the parenchymal airways and improving airway conductance. This is unlike the situation after lobectomy which does not confer these important increases in airway conductance because

**Table 8.4 Inclusion/exclusion guidelines for lung volume reduction surgery**

---

*Inclusion criteria*
Patients on optimal medical therapy
Severe intractable breathlessness caused by emphysema/hyperinflation
Diagnosis of emphysema on CT and chest X-ray (plus tests below)
Preferably heterogeneous disease with 'target areas'

Age less than 75 years
Non-smoking (check urinary nicotine)
Able to understand risk/benefit

Physiological/functional measurements (see Brenner *et al.*, 1996)

Spirometry and lung volumes
    $FEV_1$ <35% predicted
    RV >250% predicted
    RV/TLC >60%

Cardiovascular function
    Normal right and left heart function

*Exclusion criteria*
Estimated life expectancy less than 2 years

    $FEV_1$ >50% predicted
    RV <150% predicted
    TLC <100% predicted
    $FEV_1$ <500 ml (Brompton Hospital)

Oxygen prescription >18 hours per day
Hypercapnia ($PaCO_2$ >6.0 kPa)
Corticosteroid requirement >10 mg prednisolone per day

*Also:*
Previous thoracotomy
Asthma
Kyphoscoliosis
Coronary artery disease
Other major medical disease, other than emphysema

---

of the simultaneous removal of conducting airways. The increased elastic recoil following LVRS is also the mechanism whereby there is a repositioning of the chest wall and diaphragm. This leads to a more optimal chest wall position which reduces the work of breathing and decreases intrinsic positive end-expiratory pressure ($PEEP_i$). Ventilatory mechanics can improve immediately following LVRS allowing early extubation (Tschernko *et al.*, 1996). Additional positive benefits may include the recruitment of alveoli previously compressed by bullae and improved ventilation–perfusion matching because of improvement in right ventricular function.

## Surgical approaches for LVRS

A variety of surgical techniques have been developed for LVRS. These are summarized below.

## Bilateral stapling lung volume reduction via a median sternotomy

This technique was popularized by Cooper *et al.* (1995). A standard median-sternotomy is used and the pleurae are opened as one-lung ventilation is commenced. The non-ventilated lung demonstrates some degree of absorption atelectasis of the healthier areas with continued hyperinflation of diseased areas. A linear stapler buttressed with bovine pericardium is then utilized to resect 20–30% of the diseased lung volume from each lung, guided by the physical appearance of the lung and previous CT studies. Chest drainage is used as a routine.

## Video-assisted thoracoscopic (VATS) stapling LVRS

The VATS approach eliminates the complications of median sternotomy. We have had a number of problems related to the breakdown of median sternotomy wounds. This is, perhaps, not surprising in this relatively elderly group of patients who are often receiving systemic steroids.

VATS does provide good access for lung volume reduction and perhaps better visualization of posterior and inferior adhesions than does median sternotomy. It can be carried out as a bilateral procedure and is now our approach of choice.

Initially all pleural adhesions are diathermied and then chosen areas of lung tissue are stapled. Individual bullae and lung blebs can be treated separately. Staples buttressed with pericardium are available but as these are expensive they are not universally applied. Routine chest drainage is employed.

## Laser therapy for bullous emphysema

Many different techniques of laser therapy have been employed to treat emphysema. Wakabayashi (1995) is a vigorous proponent of this treatment, but his views are not universally accepted. The anaesthetic implications of thoracoscopic laser ablation of bullous emphysema have been described by Barker *et al.* (1993).

The laser can be applied to the lung surface either as an open procedure or as a VATS technique. The bullae and emphysematous areas then appear to shrink at the lung surface. Bilateral procedures are not usually undertaken as there is a significant inflammatory response.

## Anaesthetic management of LVRS

The anaesthetic management of LVRS has been reviewed by Conacher (1997). The principles we currently adopt are summarized below.

## Pre-operative preparation

All selected patients undergo an intensive rehabilitation and exercise programme. Medical treatment is optimized.

## Pre-medication

This is omitted.

### Monitoring and vascular access

As for major lung resection. A pulmonary artery catheter provides further useful information.

### Induction and maintenance of anaesthesia

- Intravenous induction with propofol
- Vecuronium or atracurium used as muscle relaxant
- Maintenance on air/oxygen mixture with either isoflurane or a propofol infusion.

We currently use an infusion of propofol as sole maintenance. This allows the use of a sophisticated ICU-type ventilator which does not have facilities to deliver inhalational agents. Isoflurane or other suitable agents are not contraindicated for this type of surgery, however. There may also be a place for the use of the new, short-acting, opioid remifentanil. In general we avoid the use of intravenous opioids because of the potential for respiratory depression.

### Analgesia

It is essential to provide good postoperative analgesia. Most authors recommend the use of thoracic or lumbar blockade with local anaesthetic agents alone or in combination with opioids. We currently use a high lumbar epidural with a bupivacaine and diamorphine mixture.

### Airway

A left-sided double lumen tube is preferred for this type of surgery. Its position is checked by fibre-optic bronchoscopy. A Univent tube is a possible alternative.

### Ventilation

Principles of management are:

- Keep the airway pressure low
- Do not use PEEP
- Pressure limit to 20 cmH$_2$O on two lungs
- Pressure limit to 30 cmH$_2$O on one-lung ventilation
- Allow permissive hypercapnia
- Allow time for expiration, e.g. I:E ratio 1:3 (or longer).

If there are signs of air trapping or hyperinflation of the ventilated lung it is safer to disconnect the patient from the ventilator to allow deflation. A period of gentle manual ventilation may be required thereafter.

### Postoperative management

Early resumption of spontaneous respiration followed by rapid extubation is advisable. This should be possible with good analgesia. The pleurae will be drained routinely but, despite meticulous surgery, air leaks are a major problem.

Opinion differs as to the management of suction to the chest drains following LVRS but air leaks are less of a problem once IPPV has been discontinued.

# Lung transplantation

The first clinically successful heart–lung transplant was carried out in Stanford in 1981. Since then single-lung, double-lung and bilateral single-lung transplantation has been developed and carried out in many centres worldwide. The supply of suitable donor lungs is now the major limiting factor in the numbers of lung transplants carried out. Newer techniques, including bilateral living-related lobar transplantation and cadaveric bilateral lobar transplantation, are being developed to overcome this problem. Xenotransplantation may also become a reality in the future. The subject of lung transplantation and its anaesthetic implications has recently been extensively reviewed by Bracken *et al.* (1997). Worldwide, single-lung transplantation is the most commonly performed operation. For the purposes of this text the anaesthetic management of single-lung transplantation is described in the following section.

# Single-lung transplantation

Single-lung transplantation is mainly undertaken for emphysema (including $\alpha_1$-antitrypsin deficiency) and idiopathic pulmonary fibrosis. A smaller number of operations are carried out for primary pulmonary hypertension. Double-lung transplantation is mainly undertaken for cystic fibrosis in children and young adults but other indications include primary pulmonary hypertension, retransplantation and congenital heart disease. In adults a significant number of double-lung transplants are also performed for emphysema.

### Selection criteria

Most lung transplant programmes have developed similar selection criteria. Recipients must have end-stage lung or pulmonary vascular disease with no other suitable treatment options. Transplantation is considered in patients with an estimated life expectancy of 12–18 months, although this is notoriously difficult to judge. Patients should also be below 60 years of age, have no other significant systemic disease and have the potential to undergo ambulatory rehabilitation. Previously steroid therapy was considered a contraindication to transplantation but most centres will now transplant those on a low dose of steroids (maximum of approximately 7.5 mg of prednisolone daily) provided there is no evidence of steroid-induced thinning of the skin, osteoporosis or myopathy. Previous thoracic surgery and a right ventricular ejection fraction of less than 25% are more controversial contraindications to surgery.

The lung function of transplant candidates is likely to be severely compromised. The $FEV_1$ may be below 20% of predicted values in patients with emphysema with a very significant (but lesser reduction) in FVC values. In patients with restrictive lung disease there will be a significant reduction in both $FEV_1$ and FVC with relative preservation of the $FEV_1$/FVC ratio. The $FEV_1$ is likely to be as low as 30% of predicted values in transplant candidates with pulmonary fibrosis. Lung function should improve dramatically following successful transplantation but very poor pre-operative lung function may forewarn of intra-operative problems, particularly in relation to one-lung anaesthesia.

## Donor organs

Donor lungs should be of suitable size with blood group compatibility with the recipient. Transplanting organs from a cytomegalovirus (CMV)-positive donor to a CMV-negative recipient should be avoided.

Suitable donors are patients less than 40 years of age who have been diagnosed as 'brain dead'. They should be haemodynamically stable, have had a short period of ventilatory support (less than 3 days), no direct pulmonary damage and no previous history of lung disease. Ideally, intended donors should have a relatively normal compliance with adequate gas exchange on 35–40% oxygen and no evidence of bacterial or fungal pulmonary infection. A worldwide shortage of donor organs has led to relaxation of donor criteria in some centres, however, so that the above criteria may now be considered too rigid. Some centres will accept donors up to 60 years of age, for example, and accept a period of ventilatory support up to 5 days.

Two methods of donor organ preservation are currently in use to allow distant procurement of the lungs. The most commonly used method entails a hypothermic plegic flush. An alternative approach, used by the Harefield (UK) group, is that of cooling the donor on cardiopulmonary bypass prior to the excision of the lungs or a heart–lung block. Cold ischaemic times should be no more than 4–6 hours with either technique.

## Operative technique

Single-lung transplantation can be carried out on the left and the right. The operation is technically easier on the left and a larger lung can be tolerated on this side because of the greater mobility of the diaphragm. An omental wrap may be used to 'protect' the bronchial anastomosis but the necessity for this remains controversial. An alternative approach to prevent ischaemia of the transplanted bronchus involves anastomosing the recipients internal mammary artery to a donor bronchial artery.

## Anaesthetic technique

### Pre-medication

No pre-medication is required in the majority of these motivated patients who may be hypoxic and on continuous oxygen therapy.

### Immunosuppression

Cyclosporin is given orally 1–2 hours before surgery and azathioprine given intravenously 1 hour prior to surgery or, alternatively, just before induction of anaesthesia. We then give 1 g of methylprednisolone intravenously when the clamp is removed following completion of the pulmonary artery anastomosis. The details of the immunosuppressive regime are likely to differ from centre to centre, however. In the postoperative period we currently rely on a combination of cyclosporin, azathioprine, prednisolone and antithymocyte globulin.

### Antibiotic therapy

Prophylactic antibiotics are given intravenously just before the induction of anaesthesia.

### Monitoring and vascular access

As for major thoracotomy.

- Vascular access should be gained under sterile conditions
- Pulmonary artery catheter and mixed venous saturation oximetry are useful. Some centres also use right ventricular ejection fraction catheters and TOE to manage right ventricular pressure and function changes appropriately.

### Airway management

A left-sided double lumen tube can be used for both right and left single-lung transplants (Boscoe, 1996). A long recipient bronchial stump remains during left lung transplant so there is room to accommodate a double lumen tube on that side. Some surgeons in the UK still prefer a right-sided tube for left lung transplantation, however, and therefore the problem of right upper lobe ventilation remains.

A Univent tube has been used as an alternative to a double lumen tube during lung transplantation and an endotracheal tube can be used for heart–lung and double-lung transplantation with tracheal anastomoses.

### Positioning

The patient is placed in a lateral position for a single-lung transplant. Access to the femoral vessels in the upper groin may be required if cardiopulmonary bypass is indicated. The pelvis is therefore tilted backwards slightly and supported on a sandbag with the upper leg straighter than usual.

### Induction and maintenance of anaesthesia

Anaesthesia is induced intravenously once intravenous and arterial lines have been inserted percutaneously under local anaesthesia and all monitoring has been established. Gross changes in haemodynamic and respiratory status should be avoided where possible by careful technique and the appropriate choice of drug therapy.

An intravenous induction with etomidate combined with an opioid such as fentanyl or alfentanil is satisfactory. Vecuronium is a suitable muscle relaxant, being devoid of histamine-releasing properties. The newer opioid remifentanil may prove useful in this field in combination with rocuronium as the muscle relaxant, but there is little data on their use in this context.

Anaesthesia can be maintained with an opioid such as fentanyl combined with a suitable volatile agent such as isoflurane in an air/oxygen mixture. A propofol infusion can be used as an alternative.

## Intra-operative management

### Fluid balance

The infusion of crystalloids should be kept to a minimum because the transplanted lung is devoid of lymphatics and cannot drain excess fluid. Mannitol is given intravenously if urine output is inadequate.

### Blood replacement

Transfused blood should be appropriate to the patient's CMV status (i.e. CMV-negative blood should be given to a CMV-negative patient). Aprotinin may help in reducing blood loss.

### Management of ventilation

Principles of management are similar to those described above for LVRS. A prolonged I:E ratio is used to allow time for expiration and hypercapnia is tolerated. Manual ventilation is indicated at times and it may also be necessary to disconnect the patient from the ventilator circuit if air trapping becomes excessive. Airway pressure should be limited to approximately 30–35 cmH$_2$O during one-lung ventilation, but this is not always feasible. Theoretically it is preferable to keep the inspired oxygen concentration as low as possible (50%) in order to prevent damage, associated with free radicals, to the donor lung. In practice 100% oxygen may be required intra-operatively in order to maintain adequate arterial oxygen saturation during one-lung ventilation. Inspired oxygen concentrations should be reduced as soon as the new lung is in circuit, however.

### Inotropic support

Dopamine is used as a continuous infusion at or above a renal dose level (Gelman, 1997). A full range of inotropic and vasodilator drugs, including adrenaline, noradrenaline, isoprenaline, milrinone, nitroglycerine and sodium nitroprusside, is prepared in bolus and infusion form for use during surgery. These drugs are particularly indicated for the treatment of right ventricular failure and pulmonary hypertension when the pulmonary artery is cross-clamped.

### Haemodynamic changes

A sudden fall in cardiac output may occur during IPPV in patients with obstructive airways disease because hyperexpansion of the lung prevents adequate venous return. This may improve if the lungs are allowed to deflate. A tension pneumothorax is another important cause of this phenomenon, which requires rapid and effective treatment.

Haemodynamically the critical point in surgery is reached when the pulmonary artery is clamped on the operative side. In patients with restrictive disease, pulmonary hypertension or a low right ventricular ejection fraction this can promote complete heart failure and circulatory collapse. Right ventricular unloading is frequently required at this point. An inspired oxygen concentration of 100% may dilate the pulmonary vasculature on the ventilated side, although nitroglycerine, isoprenaline and phosphodiesterase inhibitors are additionally beneficial in this respect. Inhaled nitric oxide is also potentially useful in this situation.

In addition to pulmonary vasodilator therapy, the right ventricle is likely to need substantial inotropic support at this stage. An inotropic dose of dopamine is a minimum requirement. Quite often an infusion of adrenaline will be required, however, to support the right heart, possibly in combination with noradrenaline to improve coronary blood flow. If these steps fail to restore haemodynamic stability and cardiac output remains low in the face of pulmonary hypertension and a low arterial saturation then cardiopulmonary bypass is indicated.

### Postoperative management

It is usual, in many centres, to change the double lumen tube to a standard endotracheal tube at the end of surgery. The surgeons can then perform fibre-optic bronchoscopy to clear the airway and inspect the anastomosis. Extubation policies differ but if early extubation is anticipated thoracic or lumbar epidural analgesia can be instituted, provided that the patient has not been recently heparinized. In practice the majority of patients are ventilated in the early postoperative period with a moderate level of PEEP to minimize the effect of reperfusion oedema. Independent lung ventilation via a double lumen tube, and two separate ventilators, may be required if hyperexpansion of the native lung causes significant compression of the transplanted lung.

### Outcome

The 1-year survival for single-lung transplantation varies between 70 and 80%. Obliterative bronchiolitis, which may be due to chronic rejection, occurs in up to 40% of single-lung recipients at 4 years. There is no effective cure for this condition, apart from retransplantation.

## Surgery of the pleura and chest wall

### Pleural disease

Patients with pleural disease commonly present to chest physicians and this complex subject has been reviewed by Vanderschueren (1995). Surgical involvement in the diagnosis and treatment of pleural disease is mainly concerned with the biopsy of the abnormal pleura, pleurectomy and pleurodesis for the treatment of pneumothorax, acute or chronic drainage of pleural effusions and the management of empyema.

Biopsy procedures, pleurectomy and pleurodesis can all be undertaken videoscopically and the principles of anaesthesia for video-assisted thoracoscopic surgery (VATS) have been discussed previously. Certain surgeons prefer to carry out some of these procedures via an open thoracotomy (albeit a small 'mini-thoracotomy'). Chronic drainage of malignant effusions and the treatment of an infected empyema may also require open surgery. These procedures and their anaesthetic implications are discussed below.

### Pleurectomy/pleurodesis

#### Indications

Pleurectomy is the operation of choice for fit patients who suffer recurrent pneumothoraces. The parietal pleura is stripped over all but the diaphragmatic surfaces of the lung. This process, combined with the ligation of obvious lung blebs or small cysts and oversuture of air leaks, is very effective in preventing further pneumothoraces. The pleural cavity is drained postoperatively and suction applied so that the lung will expand and adhere to the chest wall. This largely eliminates the possibility of a pneumothorax in the future.

Pleurodesis is a lesser operation carried out in patients with malignant disease or an underlying medical condition which makes it less likely that they will tolerate pleurectomy. Physical pleurodesis, the abrasion of both pleural surfaces with a gauze swab, can be carried out through a small incision. More often iodized talc is insufflated at thoracoscopy. This substance is highly irritant and it sets up an inflammatory reaction and promotes the formation of pleural adhesions.

Patients with cystic fibrosis are a special case (Walsh and Young, 1995). Pneumothorax is rare in children with cystic fibrosis but the incidence increases in adolescents and may occur in up to 20% of adults. Pneumothorax usually complicates severe disease and is often preceded by an infective exacerbation. Conservative management with intercostal drainage often fails in these patients and therefore a number are referred for surgery. An attempt is made to treat their problem locally because an extensive pleurectomy or pleurodesis can prejudice their chances of a successful lung transplant in later life. Specific lung air leaks and apical blebs are sutured or stapled and a pleurodesis is carried out around the leak site. This is usually done via a mini-thoracotomy, but may be possible thoracoscopically.

#### Patient characteristics

Spontaneous pneumothorax commonly occurs in:

- Young fit adults
- Tall and thin subjects
- More frequently in males and smokers.

Secondary pneumothorax occurs in:

- Chronic bronchitis and emphysema
- Cystic fibrosis
- TB
- Lung cancer.

## Risk factors

In patients with a spontaneous pneumothorax risk mainly relates to the problem of pneumothorax during anaesthesia:

- Size of the pneumothorax will increase with uptake of the soluble gas nitrous oxide
- IPPV may create a tension pneumothorax
- Both of the above are unlikely with a functioning chest drain *in situ*
- It is safer to drain a significant pneumothorax pre-operatively (a minor air space is usually tolerated).

## Monitoring/ vascular access

As for major thoracotomy.

## Positioning

Pleurectomy is usually carried out in the lateral thoracotomy position through an antero-lateral incision. For VATS pleurectomy the upper arm may be placed in a raised support to aid surgical access.

## Airway and ventilatory management

It is safer to avoid nitrous oxide and ventilatory pressures are kept to a minimum. There is always the potential for a pneumothorax to occur on the non-operative side because of bilateral disease. Endotracheal intubation may be satisfactory for the open procedure if there is either no pneumothorax present currently or if a functioning drain is in place. In practice many surgeons will expect the facility of one-lung ventilation at times and a double lumen tube is mandatory for the endoscopic technique or if there is a large air leak present. A left tube is satisfactory for either a right or left thoracotomy. Air leaks will be tested for towards the end of the procedure (as for lobectomy – Chapter 7) and chest drains will be re-inserted for postoperative management.

## Anaesthetic technique

A standard anaesthetic approach is satisfactory with an intravenous induction, neuromuscular blockade with vecuronium and maintenance with isoflurane in an air/oxygen mixture. Total intravenous anaesthesia with propofol would be equally satisfactory.

An extensive pleurectomy is a potent source of pain and pleurodesis is not benign in this respect. It is essential therefore to provide adequate analgesia by way of intravenous opioid drugs or epidural analgesia.

Bleeding can be a problem after an extensive pleurectomy, particularly if the pleura is diseased, and therefore we prefer not to give NSAIDs.

We tend not to use epidural techniques in febrile patients or patients with cystic fibrosis who may well have systemic infection at the time of surgery. This latter group undergo a lesser procedure as described above and, despite their poor lung function, they can be managed conventionally with intravenous opioids. However, some of the patients with cystic fibrosis may be in such a poor state pre-operatively, in relation to sputum retention and respiratory function, that they will benefit from a period of postoperative ventilation.

### Postoperative management

It is generally possible and desirable to re-establish spontaneous respiration in the majority of patients.

Patients after bilateral pleurectomy (now unlikely as an open procedure) may need a period of postoperative ventilation as may patients with generalized lung disease (e.g. cystic fibrosis – discussed above).

## Drainage of empyema and decortication

An empyema or infected effusion within the pleural space occurs most commonly as a complication of an infective process in the underlying lung, for example pneumonia, lung abscess or TB. Empyema can also occur after lung resection and may be associated with a bronchopleural fistula (i.e. post-pneumonectomy space infection). It may also occur after lobectomy particularly if the remaining lobe or lobes have not expanded sufficiently to fill the hemithorax.

Even if an empyema can be sterilized with antibiotics the thick exudate may not absorb but will fibrose and restrict lung movement.

The most common cause of empyema is still an underlying pneumonia and we seem to be seeing more children with this condition who are referred for chest drainage and often proceed to decortication.

Adequate drainage of a post-pneumonic empyema can usually be achieved via an intercostal drain inserted under local anaesthetic. Chronic empyemas and those following surgery may pose a more difficult drainage problem. The exact site of a loculated empyema requires defining on a CT scan. These patients also require general anaesthesia for bronchoscopy to exclude a BPF. This also allows adequate drainage of the space, with the possibility of rib resection, which is unpleasant and difficult to perform under local anaesthesia.

### Anaesthetic considerations – drainage of chronic empyema

These patients may be in poor condition because of their underlying disease and superimposed sepsis. They will generally tolerate light general anaesthesia, however, and improve symptomatically once the collection of pus has been drained. Following bronchoscopy an endotracheal tube may be inserted but a straightforward procedure can be managed with a mask or layngeal mask airway (LMA) with the patient breathing spontaneously. If a BPF is revealed at bronchoscopy endobronchial intubation will be necessary to isolate the sound lung against contamination with infected material from the empyema space.

## Decortication

A thick fibrous layer forms around the lung as a result of empyema, haemothorax or some types of sterile inflammatory effusion. This will need to be removed surgically if the lung is to expand and move relatively freely on that side.

Decortication or removal of this fibrinous layer is usually carried out through a small thoracotomy which permits dissection of the cortex from the visceral surface of the lung. Tissue planes are difficult to define, however, and there is often parietal involvement which also has to be cleared surgically.

### Anaesthetic considerations – decortication of empyema

The anaesthetic principles discussed for pleurectomy can be applied to decortication of empyema, taking into account the poor condition of patients with chronic sepsis.

A double lumen tube is used to provide one-lung anaesthesia where appropriate and is mandatory if a BPF is present. More often manual ventilation is used to hyperinflate the lung on the operative side so that the surgeon can dissect the abnormal cortex away from the lung.

Bleeding from the surface of the lung and air leak are the main intra- and postoperative problems.

## Chronic drainage of malignant pleural effusions

Patients with a persistent malignant pleural effusion can be palliated by chemical (talc) pleurodesis, provided the underlying lung will expand to fill the hemithorax. The pleurodesis will cause the lung to adhere to the chest wall and prevent further pleural fluid collecting. This procedure is usually carried out by a VATS technique.

If the lung will not expand to fill the chest, usually because of the underlying malignant process, a pleuro-peritoneal (Denver) shunt is inserted. The shunt drains pleural fluid into the peritoneum via a one-way valve, which is inserted subcutaneously in the lower chest wall, with an outlet into the abdomen. Postoperatively the patient massages the valve at regular intervals in order to aid forward flow of the fluid.

An anesthetic technique similar to that described for pleurectomy is satisfactory. The main concern will be the patient's pre-operative condition and the likely effect of the operation on respiratory function.

Many of the patients will be dyspnoeic pre-operatively and although the majority will improve, once a large effusion (often 1–2 L) has been drained, this is not always the case. Tumour invasion of the thoracic cage causes a mechanical restriction to respiration. This can be exacerbated when the underlying diseased lung adheres to the chest wall after pleurodesis. It may also remain the most important factor, combined with the deleterious effect of anaesthesia on lung function, after the insertion of a shunt.

## Surgery of the chest wall

### Correction of sternal deformity (pectus excavatum/carinatum)

Pectus excavatum and pectus carinatum (pigeon chest) are the two main categories of chest wall deformity presenting for surgery. The physiological sequelae of these deformities are usually trivial and correction is carried out almost exclusively for cosmetic reasons.

Pectus excavatum is the more common abnormality and consists of a concavity of the anterior chest wall of varying severity, usually in the lower two-thirds of the sternum. Patients are often in their late adolescence when they present for surgery.

Surgery involves meticulous dissection of the costal cartilages and mobilization of the sternum, which may be supported in its new position with a metal strut or bar.

### Anaesthetic considerations – correction of pectus excavatum/carinatum

Anaesthetic management is uncomplicated. General anaesthesia and IPPV via an endotracheal tube is entirely satisfactory and spontaneous ventilation can be re-established in the immediate postoperative period.

The major problem with the operation is that it produces a considerable amount of postoperative pain in a vulnerable group of patients. Effective analgesia is therefore essential. We advocate the use of epidural analgesia therefore, except in the unlikely event of a specific contraindication.

### Chest wall resection

Chest wall resection is occasionally required along with pulmonary resection for the treatment of lung cancer. This is undertaken only if the spread of tumour is localized and there is no evidence of distant spread. Occasionally primary chest wall tumours (e.g. sarcoma) are treated surgically.

### Anaesthetic considerations – chest wall resection

Anaesthesia can be conducted as for any major thoracotomy.

Postoperative pain control is difficult and respiratory function is impaired, particularly if lung is also resected. Resection of the posterior chest wall, particularly that covered by the scapula, does not lead to such instability as when large areas of the anterior chest wall are excised. Insertion of a chest wall prosthesis provides greater stability in the majority of cases, to prevent gross paradoxical movement, but this is obviously not perfect. Respiratory failure and sputum retention is therefore more common than following routine lung resection.

We often electively ventilate these patients until the day after surgery. This provides a stable period when secretions can be suctioned directly, analgesia optimized and spontaneous respiration gradually re-established with the aid of pressure-support ventilation.

We do not use epidural analgesia if there is a likelihood of extensive dissection around the head of ribs, near the spinal column. This can, very rarely, impair the blood supply to the spinal cord and we prefer not to be implicated as a possible cause of such an event.

## Surgery and anaesthetic management of mediastinal tumours

Mediastinal tumours are rare but inevitably present at thoracic centres for diagnostic biopsy or resection. Mediastinal masses presenting in the anterior, middle and posterior mediastinum are detailed in Table 8.5.

**Table 8.5 Mediastinal masses**

---

Anterior mediastinum
  Thymic masses
  Teratomas (germ cell tumours)
  Thyroid masses
  Lymphomas

Middle mediastinum
  Lymphomas
  Bronchial cysts
  Pericardial cysts

Posterior mediastinum
  Neurogenic tumours
    Neurofibromas
    Neurilemmomas
    Ganglioneuromas
    Meningoceles/myelomeningoceles – rare

---

From Robertson and Muers (1995)

Major anaesthetic difficulties chiefly arise in the management of anterior mediastinal tumours. These include thymic masses, retrosternal thyroid, teratomata (germ cell tumours) and lymphomas. Thymectomy for myasthenia gravis is discussed later in this chapter. The anaesthetic management of anterior mediastinal tumours is summarized below.

## Surgery for anterior mediastinal tumours

Patients with anterior mediastinal tumours usually present for biopsy initially via mediastinoscopy or mediastinotomy. A number of patients will then receive appropriate chemotherapy (e.g. for lymphoma) or radiotherapy, but a proportion will require resection of their tumours. The anaesthetic implications of biopsy and resection are the same but the risks are probably greater for the more major surgical procedure.

### Risk factors

The major problems encountered are:

- Airway obstruction – extrinsic compression by tumour
- Compression of intrathoracic vascular structures (e.g. SVC and pulmonary artery)
- Effects of previous radiotherapy and chemotherapy. (Patients could have previously received bleomycin which may affect lung function)
- Major intra-operative bleeding
- Section of phrenic and recurrent laryngeal nerves at surgery.

### Pre-operative assessment

Patients with mediastinal tumours are often in a younger age group than those with lung cancer but require a similar pre-operative 'work-up'. Further investigations will depend to some extent on symptomatology, although all these patients would undergo routine CT scanning. Guidelines for further investigation prior to anaesthesia are:

#### Respiratory symptoms – cough, dyspnoea, orthopnoea

CT or MRI scan of airway.
   Lung function tests with flow-volume loop.
   Anterior mediastinal tumours can cause quite marked compression of the trachea and main bronchi. It is remarkable that the patient can breathe through these narrowed airways. Unfortunately, after anaesthesia for even minor biopsy procedures, this ability to maintain an airway is often lost.

#### SVC obstruction

CT or MRI scan indicated.
   This physical sign is also a warning to place intravenous lines in the lower body prior to surgery – continuity from the SVC to the heart may be lost temporarily during surgery if it is necessary to clamp the SVC.

#### Cyanosis with reasonable lung function/presence of PA murmur

This may forewarn of pulmonary artery occlusion by tumour.

- CT and/or MRI scan indicated
- Echocardiography useful
- Consider angiography.

### Premedication

Omit in airway obstruction.

### Monitoring/vascular access

- As for major thoracotomy
- Insert arterial line under local anaesthetic before induction
- Additional venous line in lower limb (femoral vein preferable) in case of major surgical disruption of the SVC.

### Airway and anaesthetic management

General anaesthesia with muscular relaxation and IPPV is a suitable technique. Major problems with the airway usually relate to external compression by tumour and this should be evaluated pre-operatively.
   To circumvent the problem:

- Pre-oxygenate the patient fully
- Splint the airway with a rigid bronchoscope following an intravenous induction and intravenous suxamethonium

- Pass a long endotracheal tube or endobronchial tube through the compression to facilitate IPPV
- Consider the use of cardiopulmonary bypass, especially in the presence of pulmonary artery obstruction (very rarely indicated).

It has been recommended that an inhalational induction is used if airway narrowing is present. An inhalational induction is extremely difficult, however, if there is gross external compression. In addition extrinsic airway compression is exacerbated with induction of anaesthesia as lung volume decreases and bronchial smooth muscle relaxes. Obstructed respiration is particularly deleterious in this respect as the trachea will flatten with the large amount of negative intrathoracic pressure created. Muscular relaxation will cause a further reduction in airway support, unless the trachea is splinted internally, because of the lack of active inspiration and the loss of chest wall tone.

We prefer to use the rigid bronchoscope as the initial airway. This can be left in place until the compression is relieved surgically but it is usually satisfactory to site a long endotracheal tube or an endobronchial tube for the surgical procedure. After biopsy procedures we have ventilated patients via an double lumen tube until chemotherapy has improved airway patency. Stenting of the tracheo-bronchial tree may also help in this situation, but this type of intervention is rarely required.

## Intra-operative management

- IPPV
- Replace blood loss – this may be substantial
- Use lowest $FIO_2$ compatible with adequate arterial oxygenation if patient has had bleomycin.

## Postoperative management

Consider mechanical ventilation for the following:
- After a long procedure
- If major nerves (e.g. phrenic) sectioned intra-operatively
- Airway patency is still a problem – for example there may be tracheomalacia present following prolonged compression
- Following biopsy the patient may not be able to maintain an airway even if he or she could just prior to anaesthesia.

# Thymectomy for myasthenia gravis

## Indications

The role of the thymus in the aetiology of myasthenia gravis remains unclear but up to 75% of patients are improved by thymectomy, and may achieve complete remission over of time. A substantial number of thymus glands removed show evidence of hyperplasia and approximately 15% incorporate a thymoma.

## Patient characteristics

There are approximately 30–50 cases of myasthenia gravis per million of population. Acquired auto-immune myasthenia gravis is the most common form of the disease and is more prevalent in females. It is characterized by a weakness and fatigue of voluntary muscles. The initial presentation is often ocular with ptosis and disturbance of vision. There is a marked reduction in acetylcholine receptors at the neuromuscular junction and up to 90% of patients have circulating antibodies to these receptors.

## Treatment

Anticholinesterase therapy is the first-line treatment, but immunosuppression with corticosteroids, azathioprine or cyclosporin may also be used. Plasmapheresis is useful in a proportion of severely ill patients.

Pyridostigmine is the anticholinesterase of choice because of its long duration of action and relative lack of muscarinic side effects such as colic or excessive salivation. Atropine may still be required to counteract these latter symptoms in some patients. Neostigmine is also used to treat myasthenia but it is shorter acting than pyridostigmine and has pronounced muscarinic side effects.

## Surgical and anaesthetic considerations

Thymectomy can be undertaken via a transcervical or suprasternal approach. A limited upper median sternotomy is usually sufficient, although a complete median sternotomy may be required for an enlarged thymus. Weakness of the respiratory muscles and inability to cough or swallow are major peri-operative problems. The management of anticholinesterase therapy, induction and maintenance of anaesthesia and the conduct of postoperative ventilation are briefly outlined below.

Eisenkraft (1987) and Baraka (1992) have reviewed this subject in detail.

## Peri-operative anticholinesterase therapy

### Pre-operative period

- Reduce anticholinesterase dosage by 20% on admission to hospital (patient sedentary – overdose possible)
- Withhold pyridostigmine on morning of operation if
  1. Respiratory weakness not a problem
  2. Vital capacity at least 1 L when dose due
- If pyridostigmine required give 1/30th the oral dose as IM injection
- Omit pre-medication if respiratory/bulbar symptoms present
- IM atropine useful to prevent excessive salivation.

### Postoperative period

- Restart anticholinesterase therapy after extubation
- Original oral regime usually satisfactory
- IM pyridostigmine can be given in appropriately reduced dosage
- Oral administration can be via nasogastric tube (also if IPPV prolonged).

## Induction and maintenance of anaesthesia

Anaesthesia can be induced intravenously in the usual way and then maintained with an inhalational agent such as isoflurane.

Intubation can be achieved without muscular relaxation in many cases. Myasthenic patients are likely to be more sensitive to the neuromuscular depressant effects of inhalational agents but this varies widely from patient to patient. After anaesthesia has been deepened with isoflurane, or other suitable agents such as sevoflurane, the larynx is sprayed with lignocaine (optional) and intubation achieved without the use of muscle relaxants. Intubation may also be possible following an initial induction dose of propofol. In practice it is often simpler to use a muscle relaxant, tailoring the type of agent and the dose to the clinical situation.

## Use of muscle relaxants

Myasthenics may be resistant to the depolarizing agent suxamethonium, however, it can be used in relatively normal dosage to produce adequate relaxation for tracheal intubation with a normal recovery time.

Suxamethonium is useful to facilitate intubation in patients with little weakness or those at risk of regurgitation. Myasthenics are sensitive to non-depolarizing agents and in the past anaesthetists have generally avoided their use. Atracurium, with its unique breakdown properties, has been used successfully to provide muscular relaxation in myasthenics, however. If neuromuscular trans-mission is monitored, reduced dosage can be employed without the need for reversal. Avoiding reversal is useful in this group of patients because they may be sensitive to the effects of anticholinesterases in the postoperative period and could therefore develop a cholinergic crisis.

Mivacurium, a non-depolarizing agent with a duration of action less than that of atracurium, may also be useful in the management of myasthenics but there is little information on its use in this situation.

## Postoperative and ventilatory management

IPPV is continued into the immediate postoperative period. The effects of anaesthesia are allowed to wear off and then spontaneous ventilation is re-established. Opioids are used in reduced dosage to provide analgesia. Pain relief should not be a problem following limited sternotomy.

Extubation is performed according to the usual principles, when the patient is awake, responsive and able to generate a negative pressure of -20 cmH$_2$O.

A few patients will require prolonged ventilation and controlled weaning with titration of oral (nasogastric) anticholinesterase therapy. Patients with a severe form of myasthenia and a previous history of respiratory failure are more likely to be in this group.

After surgery, the need for maintenance therapy with anticholinesterases may be decreased or absent. Edrophonium, the very short-acting anticholinesterase, can be used (in doses of 10 mg) to differentiate weakness caused by either too small or too large a dose of anticholinesterase. It will improve the situation with too small a dose and worsen the picture with too large a dose. This type of pharmacological investigation is rarely necessary, however.

## Myasthenic syndrome

A myopathy with features resembling myasthenia gravis was reported in association with malignant disease in the 1950s. This is named the Eaton Lambert syndrome after the authors who described the electromyographic features.

### Aetiology

This condition is usually associated with small cell carcinoma of the bronchus but does occur with other neoplasms. There is now evidence of an autoimmune basis for the myasthenic syndrome with the discovery of antibodies to cationic calcium channels at the motor nerve terminal, as distinct from the antibodies to acetylcholine receptors found at the neuromuscular junction in myasthenia gravis.

The clinical features of the myasthenic syndrome and its differentiation from myasthenia gravis is shown in Table 8.6.

### Anaesthetic implications

The majority of patients with small cell lung cancer are usually inoperable at presentation and therefore rarely undergo lung resection. They may, however, present for bronchoscopy and mediastinoscopy.

In general they should be managed in a similar way to myasthenics. A greater effort should be made to avoid muscle relaxants, however, because all voluntary muscles are vulnerable.

If a conventional dose of muscle relaxant is given to a patient with myasthenic syndrome, either inadvertently or because the condition has not been formally

**Table 8.6 Differing features of myasthenia gravis and the myasthenic syndrome**

| Myasthenic syndrome | Myasthenia gravis |
|---|---|
| *Clinical features* | |
| Occurs mainly in elderly men. There is weakness and fatiguing of proximal limb muscles and tendon reflexes are reduced or absent. There is a temporary increase in strength of weakened muscles in response to exercise | More common in women. Mean age at onset 26 years. Initial symptoms of muscle weakness usually relate to ocular, oropharyngeal and limb muscle groups |
| *Response to muscle relaxants*
Sensitivity to both non-depolarizing and depolarizing drugs | Sensitive to non-depolarizing drugs
Resistant to depolarizing drugs |
| *Anticholinesterase therapy*
Poor response | Good response |
| *Pathological features*
Associated with small cell carcinoma of the lung | Thymoma present in 20–25% of cases |

recognized, it is wiser to ventilate the patient postoperatively and wait for the effect to wear off. Large doses of anticholinesterases are unlikely to be of use and may worsen the situation.

The aminopyridine group of drugs, which increase the release of acetylcholine at the neuromuscular junction, are now used orally to treat the myasthenic syndrome. In particular, 3,4-diaminopyridine is used to treat the syndrome and may also enhance the effects of anticholinesterases in patients given a non-depolarizing muscle relaxant.

## Surgery of the airway

### Tracheal resection

#### Indications

Trauma, previous tracheostomy and prolonged endotracheal intubation are the usual causes of benign strictures which present for tracheal resection. These are fortunately rare. A variety of discrete malignant tumours may also be treated by resection of the trachea but these are even more uncommon.

#### Risk factors and evaluation

The main problems of anaesthesia obviously relate to airway obstruction. The site and extent of tracheal narrowing are evaluated from the clinical history, pulmonary function tests (particularly the flow–volume loop) and a penetrated chest X-ray. More precise information can be obtained from a CT or MRI scan. Bronchoscopy may have been undertaken at an earlier stage to evaluate the stricture and facilitate bouginage or even the placement of a temporary tracheal stent.

#### Pre-medication

The majority of patients tolerate light pre-operative sedation with oral temazepam. Respiratory depressant drugs are omitted in those with severe obstruction.

#### Monitoring

As for major thoracic surgery. Place arterial line under local anaesthesia before induction.

Central venous lines should not be placed in the neck because they are likely to impinge on the site of surgery.

#### Positioning

Surgery on the upper trachea is performed via a cervical incision. A limited mediansternotomy may be required for lower stenoses. Right thoracotomy is required for access to the distal trachea and for carinal resection, and this is carried out via a lateral thoracotomy.

For upper tracheal surgery the patient is in the supine position with a sandbag under the shoulders. The head is then extended as far back as safety permits whilst held in a stabilizing head ring. Once the tracheal resection has been carried out the sandbag is removed and the head is flexed to take tension off, as the anastomosis is fashioned.

## Anaesthetic technique: airway and ventilatory management

### Induction

Pre-oxygenation followed by an intravenous induction and the administration of suxamethonium is a satisfactory induction technique for the majority of patents with a moderate stenosis.

In theory an inhalational induction should be used in those with more severe obstruction but in practice these patients rarely present for elective tracheal resection. They are much more likely to have had a procedure, such as bouginage, stent or T-tube insertion, to alleviate their stenosis at an earlier stage (see sections on bronchoscopy and tracheobronchial stent insertion – also this chapter).

### Management of ventilation

The stricture is examined at bronchoscopy. In the majority of cases some form of tracheal intubation is possible.

#### High tracheal lesion/moderate stenosis
A small, long endotracheal tube (e.g. 5.0–6.0) is passed distally to provide ventilation beyond the stenosis.

#### Mid to lower tracheal lesion/moderate stenosis
An endotracheal tube placed above the obstruction may provide satisfactory ventilation provided the stenosis is only moderate.

#### Severe tracheal stenosis
It may be necessary to pass a paediatric bronchoscope through a severe stenosis in order to dilate the stricture and allow passage of a small endotracheal tube. Very rarely it may be necessary to continue ventilation through the bronchoscope until a distal airway is established surgically. The use of HFJV or Venturi ventilation via a catheter may also be considered at this stage. It is vitally important that provision is made to allow egress of gas during exhalation, however, and these techniques are extremely risky in this situation. As alluded to above this is an unlikely scenario prior to elective tracheal resection.

Finally, cardiopulmonary bypass, established under local anaesthesia is an alternative approach to the provision of oxygenation during resection of severe and complex strictures, particularly those involving the carina. This technique carries a high risk of bleeding associated with heparinization and is not favoured by the majority of experienced surgeons.

## Intra-operative management of the airway

Once the initial airway is established anaesthesia can be maintained with an inhalational agent in oxygen or an air/oxygen mixture. A propofol infusion would also be appropriate. IPPV can be used following the administration of vecuronium or atracurium in those patients whose obstruction has been satisfactorily bypassed.

### Mid-tracheal lesions

The stricture is identified and the trachea mobilized above and below. The trachea is then transected below the stricture and a sterile, armoured endotracheal tube is inserted into the distal segment by the surgeon. Ventilation and anaesthesia are continued via an anaesthetic circuit connected to this second tube. We often use a separate Bain circuit for this purpose as its coaxial configuration is less bulky than conventional tubing.

The original tracheal tube is withdrawn proximally but left with its tip through the cords so that it can be advanced at a later stage. Some surgeons place a strong suture in the tip of this tube so that it can be guided back into place when required. The stricture can then be resected and the posterior anastomosis between the upper and lower tracheal segments fashioned whilst the armoured tube is retracted laterally or forwards. At this stage it is necessary to remove the sandbag from under the patient's shoulders and flex the neck in order to allow the ends of the trachea to be approximated with minimal tension.

The armoured tube is withdrawn once the posterior anastomosis has been completed and the original tube is advanced into the distal trachea, over the anastomosis, with its tip guided by the surgeon. Ventilation is continued via this tube whilst the anterior portion of the tracheal suture line is completed.

### Lower trachea or carinal lesions

The above technique works well for lesions of the mid and upper trachea and its simplicity has much to recommend it over more complex HFJV methods of ventilation.

The tracheal tube method of ventilation can be modified for use when the obstruction is in the lower trachea or carinal region but it may be necessary to directly intubate one or even both main bronchi. The use of HFJV or simpler Venturi ventilation via relatively fine catheters, which are less likely to obstruct upper lobe bronchi, provides better surgical access in these circumstances. Soiling of the lungs with blood is a potential problem with this technique as is the aerosol of blood produced. These catheters may also be difficult to keep in place. The relative merits of these various techniques have been discussed by Young-Beyer and Wilson (1988).

## Postoperative management

In the majority of patients spontaneous respiration is re-established in order to avoid the undesirable effects of prolonged intubation and positive-pressure ventilation on the tracheal suture line. A strong suture is used between the patient's chin and chest wall in order to keep the head flexed, thereby taking tension off the tracheal anastomosis. There have been isolated reports of serious spinal cord damage caused by overzealous flexion of the neck in these circumstances. This technique should therefore regarded as a means of preventing excessive and sudden extension of the neck, rather than a way of creating excessive flexion.

## Surgery of the oesophagus

In a book of this nature it is difficult to describe in detail the anaesthetic management for all forms of oesophageal surgery. In general, however, many of the principles of anaesthesia for lung resection can be applied to oesophageal surgery. General pre-operative assessment is similar, although there are specific features of oesophageal pathology, such as obstruction or the presence of a hiatus hernia, which have important additional consequences. The principles of general anaesthesia, one-lung ventilation and postoperative management for lung resection are equally applicable to major oesophageal surgery.

Surgery of the oesophagus in adults is mainly concerned with the management of reflux syndromes (i.e. hiatus hernia repair) and the treatment of oesophageal carcinoma. Surgery is carried out less frequently for other conditions such as benign stricture, diverticulum and achalasia of the oesophagus. The majority of patients will undergo oesophagoscopy prior to definitive surgery.

### Implications of oesophageal disease

Patients with reflux syndromes are usually in a younger age group than those with carcinoma. The major, and often the only, problem in the former group is reflux of gastric acid and food residues. In the latter (carcinoma) group there may be the sequelae of dysphagia combined with significant concomitant disease. Reflux and the aspiration of food residue from above a malignant stricture cannot be ruled out, however.

### Reflux syndromes, hiatus hernia, achalasia

The oesophagus is a muscular tube which runs from the pharynx to the stomach. The cricopharyngeus muscle closes off the pharynx and acts as an upper oesophageal sphincter but the lower oesophageal sphincter (LOS) is the major barrier preventing reflux from the stomach into the lower oesophagus.

The LOS is an area of circular muscle fibres 2–5 cm long which are innervated via the parasympathetic system. In normal subjects the LOS extends above and below the diaphragm and its pressure increases in response to an elevation of intra-abdominal pressure, thereby maintaining a barrier between stomach and oesophagus. This mechanism is deranged by oesophageal abnormalities such as hiatus hernia and it is also affected by drug therapy and diet (Table 8.7).

Induction of anaesthesia followed by the administration of muscle relaxants is particularly likely to lead to regurgitation of stomach contents in patients with LOS dysfunction, unless appropriate precautions are taken.

Achalasia of the oesophagus is a generalized disorder of oesophageal motility characterized by incoordinate or absent peristalsis. The LOS tone in these patients is normal or slightly elevated. The oesophagus gradually dilates,

**Table 8.7 Effects of drugs and diet on lower oesophageal sphincter tone**

| Increase | Decrease | No change |
| --- | --- | --- |
| Metoclopramide | Atropine | Propranolol |
| Domperidone | Glycopyrrolate | Oxprenolol |
| Prochlorperazine | Dopamine | Cimetidine |
| Cyclizine | Ganglion blockers | Ranitidine |
| Edrophonium | Thiopentone | Omeprazole |
| Neostigmine | ß-agonists | Atracurium |
| Histamine | Halothane | |
| Suxamethonium | Enflurane | |
| Pancuronium | Opioids | |
| Metoprolol | Alcohol | |
| Adrenergic agonists | Caffeine | |
| Antacids | | |
| Cisapride | | |

Adapted from Aitkenhead (1987)

however, and becomes grossly enlarged being filled with food residues and secretions. These patients are at high risk from aspiration at induction of anaesthesia and should be treated accordingly. They often suffer repeated episodes of aspiration into the lungs prior to surgery and this may result in bronchopneumonia and even lung abscess. The oesophagus is emptied of its contents via a rigid oesophagoscope prior to surgical treatment (Heller's operation/oesophageal myotomy).

**Table 8.8 Measures to prevent or mitigate the effects of acid aspiration prior to oesophageal surgery**

*Drug therapy*

*Proton pump inhibitor*
  Omeprazole (or other suitable drug)
  Give the night before surgery

*$H_2$ receptor antagonist*
  Ranitidine, cimetidine or other suitable alternative
  Give the night before and 2 hours before surgery
  IV administration with dysphagia

*Metoclopramide*
  Stimulates gastric emptying and small intestinal transit
  Give with pre-medication

*Antacids*
  Sodium citrate (30 ml of a 0.3 molar solution) orally
  Give 30 min prior to surgery
  Clear fluid; does not obscure view at oesophagoscopy

*Physical methods*
  Rapid sequence induction
  Cricoid pressure
  Slight head-up tilt

Prevention of reflux at induction of anaesthesia for oesophageal surgery is predominantly by means of a rapid sequence induction, with cricoid pressure applied to occlude the oesophageal lumen. This, plus measures that can be taken to reduce gastric acid secretion and promote gastric emptying, are summarized in Table 8.8.

# Carcinoma of the oesophagus

Severe progressive dysphagia is the characteristic symptom of oesophageal carcinoma at any level. A high proportion of patients have inoperable lesions at presentation, however, and palliative treatment is all that can be offered.

Patients presenting for oesophagoscopy and potentially oesophagectomy, may be dehydrated, debilitated and generally malnourished as a consequence of dysphagia. Anaemia and hypoalbuminaemia are not uncommon. In addition many of these patients are elderly smokers and therefore have many cardiovascular and respiratory risk factors in common with lung resection candidates. Oesophageal carcinoma is also associated with a high alcohol intake.

Every effort should be made to improve nutrition pre-operatively, particularly if an extensive surgical resection is planned. A high calorie/high protein liquid diet may be tolerated if the oesophagus is not completely obstructed by tumour. Alternatively a percutaneous endoscopic gastrostomy (PEG) can be performed to provide a route for direct enteral feeding.

# Oesophagoscopy

## Indications

Oesophagoscopy is used to visualize the lower pharynx and oesophagus. It provides access for endoscopic examination and biopsy of tumours, removal of foreign bodies, dilatation of strictures and palliative intubation of malignant obstruction. A rigid oesophagoscope, inserted under general anaesthesia, gives a good view of the oesophageal mucosa and is large enough to allow the passage of large biopsy forceps and dilators. The rigid oesophagoscope requires careful handling by an experienced surgeon, however, as its use is potentially hazardous.

The flexible fibre-optic oesophagoscope can be used with only topical analgesia and light sedation and is passed down the oesophagus more easily than the rigid instrument. It can also be advanced to view the stomach and duodenum.

## Risk factors

The main risk factors of this procedure relate to regurgitation/acid aspiration at induction of anaesthesia and concomitant medical disease.

## Premedication

Light oral premedication with temazepam is usually a satisfactory. If the patient is debilitated or has dysphagia this can be omitted. We do not feel that an anticholinergic agent is mandatory prior to oesophagoscopy but antacid prophylaxis is prescribed where appropriate (Table 8.8).

### Monitoring/vascular access

Monitoring requirements are similar to bronchoscopy with an ECG, non-invasive blood pressure measurement and pulse oximetry as a minimum. End-tidal gas analysis is also useful. Intra-operative dysrhythmias are not uncommon as the oesophagoscope is advanced and they also occur during balloon dilatation of the oesophagus. These are usually benign and do not require treatment, but nevertheless the ECG needs to be monitored closely throughout the procedure.

### Positioning

Oesophagoscopy is carried out with the patient in a supine position. If this is carried out on an operating table the head can easily be extended to facilitate passage of the rigid oesophagoscope. We take steps to protect the patient's eyes and take care not to damage the upper incisors as the rigid scope is introduced into the mouth and advanced down the oesophagus. The comments made earlier in this chapter concerning bronchoscopy and the patient with an unstable neck apply equally to oesophagoscopy.

### Anaesthetic technique/airway management

#### *Induction*

An intravenous induction with propofol is satisfactory in the majority of cases, but dosage should be kept to a minimum in elderly and/or debilitated patients. A rapid sequence induction, with the application of cricoid pressure, is undertaken in those patients at risk of aspiration.

#### *Muscular relaxation*

It is important to establish complete muscular relaxation so that the oesophago-scope can be safely passed through the cricopharyngeal sphincter at the inlet to the oesophagus. Suxamethonium is still the best drug to use if cricoid pressure is to be employed, and this can be repeated in incremental doses for a short procedure. For a longer procedure atracurium or mivacurium can be given to extend muscular relaxation. Alternatively, these latter drugs can be given from the outset if there is no risk of aspiration.

#### *Intubation*

Endotracheal intubation is carried out with an armoured oral tube one size smaller than normal. The tracheal cuff may need to be deflated slightly to allow passage of the oesophagoscope through cricopharyngeus.

#### *Maintenance of anaesthesia*

Anaesthesia is usually maintained with an oxygen/air or an oxygen/nitrous oxide inspired gas mixture combined with a suitable inhalational agent. A propofol infusion is also satisfactory.

It can be useful to employ manual ventilation during the procedure in order to anticipate and control coughing, which can lead to oesophageal damage.

### Postoperative management/complications

At the end of the procedure muscular relaxation is reversed, as necessary, and the patient extubated when awake in a lateral position.

A postoperative chest X-ray is mandatory. This is checked for signs of oesophageal rupture, including surgical emphysema, pneumothorax, pneumomediastinum and pneumoperitoneum, before oral fluids are commenced.

## Surgery for carcinoma of the oesophagus

### Indications

Approximately 50% of oesophageal tumours are unresectable at presentation and of those tumours considered operable long-term results remain depressing in most western series with 5-year survival as low as 10%.

The majority of tumours are in the middle and lower thirds of the oesophagus and these can be resected via a left thoraco-abdominal approach. Stomach or colon is then mobilized and brought up to restore the continuity of the alimentary tract. Oesophagogastrectomy may be required if the stomach is involved. Operative mortality remains high for these procedures (as high as 10–20% in some series) and long-term survival depends on the extent of nodal spread at the time of surgery.

Although the left thoraco-abdominal approach is popular for the lower oesophagus a variety of different surgical techniques may be used including a supine abdominal approach followed by a right thoracotomy for middle third tumours and a combined approach involving laparotomy, right thoracotomy and a cervical incision for upper third tumours. The sequence of the planned procedure should be fully discussed with the surgeon before operation as this will have a major bearing on positioning of the patient and the sites of vascular access.

A substernal gastric bypass may be performed as an alternative palliative procedure and endoscopic techniques have been developed for oesophageal resection. In general, endoscopic techniques are still not considered the most appropriate approach for curative cancer surgery.

### Patient characteristics

These patients are often elderly smokers (male>female), as described above, with the additional systemic and metabolic consequences of dysphagia. The risk factors for operation relate to the major nature of the surgery in a group of patients who may range from ASA status II– IV, in terms of their pre-existing medical condition.

The pre-operative assessment of these patients is similar to that described for lung resection in Chapter 6. Postoperatively anastomotic leaks are a major and significant source of morbidity and mortality.

## Premedication

Light, oral, premedication is prescribed in the majority of patients.

Antibiotic prophylaxis, commonly cephalosporin and metronidazole, is commenced immediately after induction of anaesthesia.

## Monitoring/vascular access

Monitoring and vascular access is usually as previously described for a major lung resection. If a high colonic anastomosis is planned via a cervical incision, however, central venous lines should not be sited in the neck.

Blood and fluid loss can be extensive during major oesophageal surgery and this should be replaced appropriately with warmed colloid and bank blood. Heat loss is very significant from the large surface area of lung and abdominal contents exposed during a thoraco-abdominal laparotomy and a convective warm air heating device is, therefore, used to maintain body temperature.

## Positioning

Positioning will depend entirely on the planned procedure. Commonly, a semi-lateral position is used to give access to the oesophagus via a left thoraco-abdominal incision.

## Airway and ventilatory management

A double lumen endobronchial tube is inserted to provide one-lung anaesthesia and facilitate surgical access to the oesophagus. In this context a left-sided tube eliminates the problem of right upper lobe ventilation, but our surgeons prefer a right-sided tube for a left thoraco-abdominal procedure. This is because they believe a left-sided tube is more likely to kink and obstruct as the left lung is retracted to allow mobilization of the oesophagus.

## Anaesthetic technique

An intravenous induction is carried out with propofol or etomidate. Cricoid pressure is applied, where necessary, in which case suxamethonium is given as the initial muscle relaxant. Otherwise a non-depolarizing agent such as pancuronium or vecuronium is used from the outset.

Epidural analgesia is extremely useful because of the pain produced by a large thoraco-abdominal incision. We prefer to establish this, immediately after induction of anaesthesia, in the high lumbar region. Intravenous opioids are widely used, however, if postoperative ventilation is planned.

## Postoperative management

Early resumption of spontaneous respiration may be satisfactory, and even preferred, after a straightforward procedure with effective epidural analgesia.

The endotracheal tube should only be removed, however, when the patient is alert and in a sitting position. This is because a conduit of stomach or colon does not provide a mechanical barrier to prevent aspiration of gut/stomach contents.

We prefer a period of postoperative ventilation for the majority of patients. Spontaneous respiration can then be resumed gradually in optimal circumstances when heat loss, fluid balance and abnormalities of gas exchange have been corrected.

# References

Aitkenhead A.R. (1987) Anaesthesia for oesophageal surgery. In *Thoracic Anaesthesia. Clinical Anaesthesiology.* (Ed. Gothard J.W.W.). Baillière Tindall, London, Vol. 1, 181–206.

Baraka A. (1992) Anaesthesia and myasthenia gravis. *Can J Anaesth;* **39:** 476–486.

Barker S.J., Clarke C., Trivedi N. *et al.* (1993) Anesthesia for thoracoscopic laser ablation of bullous emphysema. *Anesthesiology;* **78:** 44–50.

Boscoe M.J. (1996) Lung and heart–lung transplantation. In *Handbook of Clinical Anaesthesia;* (Eds Goldstone J.C. and Pollard B.J.). Churchill Livingstone, London, Vol. 23, 467–469..

Bracken C.A., Gurkwoski M.A. and Naples J.J. (1997) Lung transplantation: historical perspective, current concepts, and anesthetic considerations. *J Cardiothorac Vasc Anesth;* **11:** 220–241.

Brenner M., Yusen R., McKenna R. *et al.* (1996) Lung volume reduction surgery for emphysema. *Chest;* **110:** 205–218.

Conacher I. (1997) Anaesthesia for the surgery of emphysema. *Br J Anaesth;* **79:** 530–538.

Cooper J.D., Trulock E.P., Triantafillou A.N. *et al.* (1995) Bilateral pneumectomy (volume reduction) for chronic obstructive pulmonary disease. *J Thorac Cardiovasc Surg;* **109:** 106–119.

Eaton L.M. and Lambert L.M. (1957) Electromyography and electrical stimulation of nerves in disease with motor units. Observations on myasthenic syndrome associated with malignant tumours. *JAMA;* **163:** 1117–1124.

Eisenkraft J.B. (1987) Myasthenia gravis and thymic surgery – anaesthetic considerations. In *Thoracic Anaesthesia. Clinical Anaesthesiology.* (Ed. Gothard J.W.W.). Baillière Tindall, London, Vol. 1, 133–162.

Gelman S. (1997) Low-dose dopamine: there is a scientific rationale. *Br J Anaesth;* **79:** 546.

Hill A.J., Feneck R.O., Underwood S.M. *et al.* (1991) The haemodynamic effects of bronchoscopy. Comparison of propofol and thiopentone with and without alfentanil. *Anaesthesia;* **46:** 266–270.

Plummer S., Hartley M. and Vaughan R.S. (1998) Anaesthesia for telescopic procedures in the thorax. *Br J Anaesth;* **80:** 223–234.

Robertson R. and Muers M. (1995) Mediastinal masses. *Medicine;* **23:** 369–371.

Tschernko E.M., Wisser W., Hofer S. *et al.* (1996) The influence of lung volume reduction on ventilatory mechanics in patients suffering from severe chronic obstructive pulmonary disease. *Anesth Analg;* **83:** 996–1001.

Vanderschueren R. (1995) Pleural disease. *Medicine;* **23:** 256–261.

Wakabayashi A. (1995) Thoracoscopic pneumoplasty in the treatment of diffuse bullous emphysema. *Ann Thorac Surg;* **60:** 936–942.

Walsh T.S. and Young C.H. (1995) Anaesthesia and cystic fibrosis. *Anaesthesia;* **50:** 614–622.

Young-Beyer P. and Wilson R.S. (1988) Anesthetic management for tracheal resection and reconstruction. *J Cardiothorac Anesth;* **2:** 821–835.

Chapter 9

# Postoperative management

In the immediate postoperative period the main concerns are to establish a satisfactory respiratory pattern, haemodynamic stability and good analgesia. This is best accomplished in a high dependency unit (HDU) with full monitoring and ventilation facilities and, most importantly, trained nursing staff.

The majority of patients will be extubated in the operating theatre once spontaneous respiration has been established. Some patients, however, will require a period of mechanical ventilation and this is discussed below.

The spontaneously breathing patient is nursed in the upright sitting position. Supplemental oxygen is supplied by face mask, preferably a fixed performance device. The invasive monitoring utilized in the operating theatre is continued in the HDU and rewarming completed via a convective warm air heating device. Initial investigations required in the first few hours are listed in Table 9.1. These include serial blood gas analyses and a portable chest X-ray. Specific points to note in the first postoperative chest X-ray are detailed in Table 9.2.

**Table 9.1 Initial postoperative investigations**

Arterial blood gas analysis and haemoglobin estimation

Serum potassium and sodium (plus urea and creatinine if NSAIDs are to be used)

Blood sugar (or BM stix estimation)

Clotting studies and platelet count – if bleeding excessive

Portable chest X-ray

**Table 9.2 Specific points to note in initial postoperative chest X-ray**

- Position of mediastinum
- Full expansion of lung fields (check right upper lobe if right-sided double lumen tube has been used)
- Evidence of pneumothorax (this should not be present if full lung expansion is achieved at the end of surgery and the chest drains are patent)
- Position of endotracheal tube – if present
- Position of central venous lines (check for pneumothorax if venous cannulation has been attempted on the non-operative side)
- Presence of any pleural fluid

## Respiratory management

### Postoperative ventilation

As discussed previously the majority of patients can be allowed to breathe spontaneously following thoracic surgery. Some patients may require a short period of mechanical ventilation whilst the effects of anaesthetic agents and opioids (intravenous or epidural) are allowed to 'wear off' rather than be abruptly antagonized with naloxone. In this group of patients we often ventilate via the double lumen tube, with the bronchial cuff deflated and/or the tube partially withdrawn into the trachea.

A further subset of patients, particularly frail elderly patients with poor lung function who have undergone extensive surgery, benefit from elective post-operative ventilation. In this latter group we change the double lumen tube to an endotracheal tube at the end of surgery and transfer the patient to the intensive care unit for a period of postoperative ventilation (often overnight). This period of ventilation allows rewarming, correction of fluid/acid–base balance, optimum recovery from intra-operative atelectasis, plus the establishment of adequate analgesia to be carried out in a controlled environment.

Intermittent positive pressure ventilation (IPPV) is established and optimized in the usual manner. Our surgeons do not worry unduly regarding the effect of positive pressure or suction on their bronchial stump anastomoses but an attempt is made to keep inflation pressures within the normal range. If necessary pressure-limited ventilation can be used.

### Chest drainage

Pleural or chest drainage is an essential part of the management of the post-thoracotomy patient. Chest drains allow the escape of air, blood or fluid from the pleural space in order to restore cardiorespiratory function by re-expansion of the lung and elimination of mediastinal shift. The essential components of a simple chest drainage system are listed in Table 9.3.

**Table 9.3 Components of a chest drainage system**

Pleural tube
　To evacuate air, blood or fluid with minimal resistance

　A 32-French gauge tube is commonly used. (With -10 cmH$_2$O suction this will allow an airflow of approximately 35–40 L per min. In practice -5 kPa is applied; approx. -50 cmH$_2$O of suction)

Underwater seal
　One-way valve to allow expulsion of air and fluid from the pleural cavity and prevent re-entry of air during inspiration

Collecting chamber
　For blood/fluid

Suction
　Usually 5 kPa
　Must be capable of clearing large volumes of air

## Chest drainage after lung resection (e.g. lobectomy)

Two chest drains are commonly inserted following lung resection (other than pneumonectomy). Classically an apical drain is used to remove air which has risen towards the apex and a basal drain collects fluid which has gravitated downwards (Fig. 9.1). An alternative, and equally effective approach, is to place anterior and posterior drains towards the apex with side holes to provide basal drainage (Fig. 9.2).

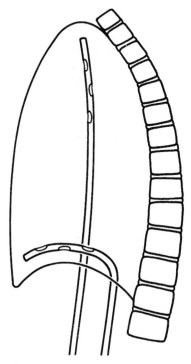

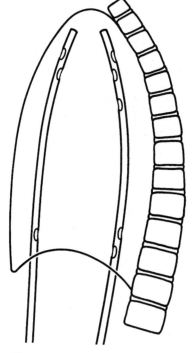

Fig. 9.1 Apical and basal chest drains. Reproduced with permission from Gothard J.W.W. (1993) *Anaesthesia for Thoracic Surgery*, 2nd edn. Blackwell Scientific Publications

Fig. 9.2 Anterior and posterior chest drains. Reproduced with permission from Gothard J.W.W. (1993) *Anaesthesia for Thoracic Surgery*, 2nd edn. Blackwell Scientific Publications

## Chest drainage after pneumonectomy

Air leak does not occur after pneumonectomy and therefore chest drainage is not mandatory. Some surgeons, therefore, close the chest without a drain if they are confident that there is no significant bleeding. If a chest drain is not inserted, air is aspirated from the pneumonectomy space at the end of operation, with the patient in a supine position. This can be done simply with a 50 ml syringe and a three-way tap connected to a long intravenous cannula placed through the chest wall. Several 100 ml of air are aspirated until there is a slight 'pull' on the syringe, indicating a negative pressure within the empty hemithorax. At this stage the mediastinum, which will have migrated towards the dependent lung during lateral thoracotomy, should be approximately central or slightly towards the side of surgery. This position can be verified crudely by feeling the position of the trachea or more accurately by inspecting the postoperative chest X-ray. Occasionally it may be necessary to aspirate further air in the postoperative period.

Some surgeons prefer to place a chest drain in all patients following pneumonectomy, particularly if there has been significant problems with haemostasis. This is usually a single basal drain (Fig. 9.3) which is left clamped but connected to an underwater seal drain. Traditionally the clamp is released for 1–2 min in every hour in order to reveal excessive blood loss and centralize the mediastinum by releasing trapped air. In spite of traditional teaching, however, a small number of surgeons leave the chest drain unclamped after pneumonectomy. This does not seem to cause excessive mediastinal shift but can lead to paradoxical mediastinal movement and less effective sputum clearance of the remaining lung.

Suction is not applied to a pneumonectomy drain under any circumstances. This will pull the mediastinum across and severely impede or totally obstruct venous return to the heart with disastrous consequences. Pneumonectomy drains

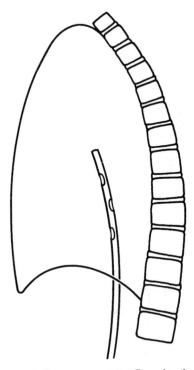

**Fig. 9.3** Basal chest drain, as used after pneumonectomy. Reproduced with permission from Gothard J.W.W. (1993) *Anaesthesia for Thoracic Surgery,* 2nd edn. Blackwell Scientific Publications

are removed the day after surgery if there is no active bleeding. This allows the pneumonectomy space to fill with exudate and fluid in the usual manner.

### Design of underwater seal drains

An underwater seal is essentially a one-way valve mechanism to allow expulsion of air and fluid out of the pleural space and to prevent re-entry of atmospheric air. Various designs of drainage bottle are made but in theory a large diameter bottle is preferable with the chest drain/connecting tube terminating only 2 cm below the water surface (Fig. 9.4). This provides minimal resistance to the escape of air but a huge inspiratory effort would be required to break the seal by drawing water into the tubing from the bottle, assuming the bottle is kept well below the patient. A large diameter collecting bottle is desirable so that the volume of water above the distal end of the submerged drainage tubing is greater than the volume of the drainage tubing from patient to bottle.

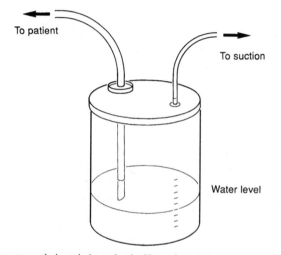

To patient

To suction

Water level

**Fig. 9.4** An underwater seal chest drainage bottle. Note: chest drainage bottles should be relatively broad, with a diameter of 14 cm or more; see text. Reproduced with permission from Gothard J.W.W. (1993) *Anaesthesia for Thoracic Surgery,* 2nd edn. Blackwell Scientific Publications

The main disadvantage of the simple system described above is that there is increasing resistance to drainage as the bottle fills with blood or fluid. This resistance to drainage is, however, largely overcome by the use of suction (Kam *et al.*, 1993).

### Suction applied to chest drains

Suction increases the pressure difference between the pleural space and the chest drain bottle by drawing air from the bottle, causing a decrease in pressure within the bottle. Suction promotes expansion of the lung and assists the escape of air or fluid from the pleural space. It also eliminates the possibility of air entering the chest. This is because even the most vigorous inspiratory effort (up to $-80\,cmH_2O$) cannot overcome the negative pressure provided by the pump combined with the negative pressure effect of gravity as a result of fluid entering the drainage tubing from the bottle placed well below the patient.

Low-pressure suction (up to $5\,kPa$ or $50\,cmH_2O$) may be applied but this must be provided via a pump that is capable of clearing large volumes of air. Modern pipeline low-pressure suction units are usually sufficient to maintain a negative pressure in the face of all but the largest air leaks. Low-pressure, low-volume devices such as the Roberts pump cannot clear large volumes of air and may act as an obstruction to drainage in the presence of a large air leak.

### Excessive or persistent air leak

The surgeon will attempt to minimize air leak following thoracotomy by suturing any small patent bronchi and by the application of diathermy to raw lung surfaces. The volume of air leak may, very rarely, be unacceptable in the immediate postoperative period and re-exploration is justified in case the lung has been transfixed by pericostal sutures. The air leak will, more commonly, lessen progressively as lung tissue expands to fill the thoracic cavity and seal the area of air leak against the chest wall. A persistent air leak after lobectomy, with the remaining lobe or lobes failing to fill the thoracic cavity, will almost inevitably lead to the production of a localized empyema cavity.

### Removal of chest drains

Chest drains are removed once they have ceased to function. From the practical point of view this means when air or fluid loss has not occurred over the preceding 12–24 hours and when the pleural space has been obliterated by adhesions as evidenced by the chest X-ray, the cessation of bubbling within the drainage bottle and the reduction of the respiratory swing of the water level.

Chest drains should be removed by a competent trained nurse. There may be some discomfort during the removal of the drains and as a result a natural tendency for patients to inspire. Removal is therefore undertaken during a Valsalva manoeuvre at full inspiration, thereby maintaining a positive intrapleural pressure and preventing influx of air. A horizontal mattress suture placed around the chest drain at the time of its insertion is tightened as the drain is removed, to prevent air entering via the wound. After removal a chest X-ray is obtained to exclude a pneumothorax.

### Sputum retention

Problems of sputum retention after thoracic surgery can be considered the norm in smokers. Smoking induces mucus gland hyperplasia and mucosal metaplasia together with impaired cilial function. Sputum retention is, therefore, to be expected after surgical trauma to the lungs is superimposed on these physiological and functional defects.

Patients with poor lung function, and particularly those whose $FEV_1$ is less than $1.0\,L$ postoperatively, cannot cough effectively enough to clear secretions. In addition, resection of the recurrent laryngeal nerve leaves the larynx incompetent preventing an adequate rise in intrathoracic pressure prior to the explosive act of coughing. Similarly, phrenic nerve damage results in paradoxical diaphragmatic movement. This also reduces the force of coughing but can be offset to some extent by plication of the diaphragm on the side of surgery. Finally, chest wall resection can cause a degree of paradoxical respiration even after the insertion of a rigid chest wall prosthesis. Secretions are likely to accumulate, therefore, in the inadequately ventilated areas of lung underlying this area.

Physiotherapy is, in the presence of adequate analgesia, an effective method of clearing retained sputum. This is largely a mechanical problem but retained secretions are likely to become infected and appropriate antibiotic cover is instituted on the basis of sputum cultures.

If these simple measures fail to solve the problem of sputum retention a mini-tracheostomy tube can be inserted through the cricothyroid membrane as a direct route for bronchial suction. This procedure, carried out under local anaesthesia, is theoretically straightforward. In unskilled hands it can lead to disaster as a result of bleeding into or around the trachea, which can only further impair arterial oxygenation. Mini-tracheostomy should not therefore be delegated to the unsupervised novice.

Continuing difficulties with sputum clearance, despite the above measures, usually leads to endotracheal intubation and mechanical ventilation. Formal tracheostomy may be required later to aid weaning from ventilation in this small group of patients.

## Respiratory failure

There is restricted ventilation and an altered pattern of breathing following thoracotomy (Entwistle *et al.*, 1991). The characteristic mechanical abnormalities result in a reduction in vital capacity, tidal volume and $FEV_1$ as well as the reduction in functional residual capacity associated with anaesthesia.

Pain is the principal inhibitor of chest wall movement, but obesity, the supine position and interstitial oedema of damaged tissue all have a restrictive effect on ventilation. As a result postoperative hypoxaemia is almost inevitable following thoracotomy and it is out of proportion to the quantity of lung removed or collapsed. Patients who are hypoxaemic pre-operatively, not surprisingly, are more likely to be so postoperatively (Table 9.4). Measures that can be adopted to minimize hypoxaemia and pulmonary complications are detailed in Table 9.5.

In addition to hypoxia, carbon dioxide retention is also a problem following thoracotomy. During the first few hours after surgery hypercarbia is common. As

**Table 9.4 Pattern of oxygenation before and after thoracic surgery: numbers of patients (out of 20) showing a particular pattern**

| Oxygen saturation pattern | Pre-op | 1st night | 2nd night | 4th night |
|---|---|---|---|---|
| Stable, not hypoxic | 11 | 2 | 3 | 5 |
| Stable, hypoxic (but improving) | 0 | 8 | 0 | 0 |
| Stable, hypoxic | 9 | 5 | 12 | 11 |
| Unstable, hypoxic | 0 | 5 | 5 | 0 |

Note: the patients who were hypoxic before surgery, not surprisingly, remained so postoperatively
(Entwistle *et al.*, 1991)

**Table 9.5 Measures to reduce pulmonary complications**

- Provision of adequate analgesia with minimal respiratory depression
- Erect or semi-erect upper body position to increase FRC
- Humidified oxygen therapy to reduce tenacity of secretions
- Regular physiotherapy
- Incentive spirometry
- Continuous positive airway pressure (CPAP) intermittently by face mask

satisfactory analgesia is established in the patient awakening from anaesthesia serial blood gas analyses are undertaken to monitor oxygenation and possible carbon dioxide retention. A raised $PaCO_2$ is not initially of great concern provided the trend of serial estimations is downwards and the patient is awake with a satisfactory respiratory pattern. We do not transfer the patient to a ward from the high dependency area until the $PaCO_2$ is approximately 7.0 kPa, or less, with a downward trend in measured values. If carbon dioxide levels are towards the upper end of this limit we keep the arterial line *in situ* and continue to monitor arterial blood gas values on the ward.

Chronic obstructive pulmonary disease (COPD) is a frequent finding in patients presenting for thoracic surgery, although this is unlikely to be severe in those scheduled for lung resection. Carbon dioxide retention and hypoxaemia secondary to alveolar hypoventilation are nevertheless particular risks in this group. Patients should therefore be monitored carefully whilst breathing a known, fixed concentration of oxygen. The bicarbonate level in a pre-operative arterial blood gas sample will provide a further guide as to what level of arterial $PaCO_2$ can be expected in these patients.

### Acute lung injury and post-pneumonectomy pulmonary oedema

From the above discussion concerning sputum retention and respiratory failure after thoracic surgery, plus the description of acute lung injury (ALI) following one-lung ventilation (Chapter 7), it will be appreciated that lung surgery combines many of the elements involved in the aetiology of acute respiratory distress syndrome (ARDS). ARDS has an overall incidence of 4–5% following lung resection and has also been termed post-pneumonectomy pulmonary oedema (PPE) in the North American literature. The term PPE also encompasses lobectomy patients, however.

Reperfusion injury has been implicated in the aetiology of ARDS after lung resection but a number of other factors are associated with this problem. Possible causes of, and contributing factors to, PPE are listed in Table 9.6. The effects of some of these factors, specifically fluid overload, hyperinflation and right ventricular failure, can be ameliorated by specific management strategies.

Fluid overload has certainly been incriminated as a cause of PPE in many studies, but by no means all. It is recommended therefore (Slinger, 1995) that fluid overload is avoided peri-operatively and that a total positive fluid balance should not exceed 20 ml/kg for the first 24 hours (including the operative period). Blood and fluid loss at operation are often difficult to estimate, however, and

**Table 9.6 Factors contributing to post-pneumonectomy pulmonary oedema**

- Fluid overload
- Damage to lymphatic drainage (surgical)
- Hyperinflation of lung intra-operatively ('volutrauma')
- Right ventricular dysfunction
- Reperfusion injury
- Cytokine release
- Oxygen toxicity

some patients may already have an element of renal dysfunction which will further deteriorate in the face of dehydration.

Hyperinflation of the lung during one-lung ventilation has also been incriminated as a factor contributing to PPE. It may be that conventional tidal volumes of 10 ml/kg during one-lung ventilation approach the levels that can cause volutrauma. This is particularly so after right pneumonectomy where damage to the left lung lymphatic drainage also has a role to play. Using lower tidal volumes in patients with high inflation pressure or abnormal pressure–volume loops (Simon, 1992; Bardoczky, 1993) may limit ventilatory damage intra-operatively. We also take care not to overinflate the lung when testing for lung air leaks and bronchial stump competence.

Right ventricular dysfunction, caused by an increased afterload as the cardiac output is channelled through a smaller pulmonary vascular bed, is common following thoracotomy. Following pneumonectomy patients have an increase in pulmonary vascular resistance of up to 30% on exercise and this is accompanied by desaturation. Post-thoracotomy patients also have an increase in right ventricular pressure in the early postoperative period which coincides with the withdrawal of supplemental oxygen. Hypercarbia contributes to an increase in pulmonary artery pressure. In high-risk patients oxygen therapy should be continued until satisfactory saturations are sustained continuously on room air. If overt right ventricular failure is suspected clinically, and confirmed by central venous pressure measurements and echocardiography, then inotropic and pulmonary vasodilator therapy is indicated.

# Cardiovascular complications and management

## Hypotension

Hypotension is not uncommon in the early postoperative period. As the patient is fully rewarmed and analgesia is established peripheral vasodilatation occurs. Our standard fluid regime of dextrose/saline solution, 1 ml/kg/hour (with potassium supplementation), is therefore inadequate at this stage. Transfusion of colloid is required in order to 'fill' the circulation. We usually use an artificial plasma expander such as a starch solution if the haemoglobin level is satisfactory and infuse this on the basis of the central venous pressure and clinical condition of the patient. It may be necessary to transfuse up to 1 L or more of colloid, but above this level a careful reappraisal of the patient's clinical status is required to avoid overtransfusion.

If hypotension persists, despite presumed adequate volume replacement, and blood loss into the drains is not excessive, hidden blood loss should be sought. Considerable amounts of blood can accumulate in a pneumonectomy space. This may or may not be revealed if the chest drain is briefly unclamped but a chest X-ray, showing a rapidly filling space, is an indication that active blood loss is continuing in those with or without a drain. Similarly, a chest X-ray may reveal sequestered clot after lobectomy.

If hypotension persists despite adequate filling it may be necessary to initiate inotropic therapy, particularly in those patients known to have pre-existing myocardial dysfunction. A urinary catheter should also be inserted at this stage if one is not already in place. If a relatively low dose of an inotrope such as dopamine or dobutamine fails to improve blood pressure, cardiac output and urine output, then investigation and treatment of the hypotension should be escalated. Placement of a Swan Ganz catheter will allow measurement of left-sided cardiac filling pressures and cardiac output. This, combined with echocardiographic assessment, will guide further management. In practice these latter steps are rarely indicated.

## Hypertension and myocardial ischaemia

Thoracic surgical patients often have concomitant cardiovascular disease as discussed in Chapter 6. Anti-anginal therapy is always continued up to and including the day of surgery and should be recommenced postoperatively. In the immediate postoperative period hypertension can occur, particularly if analgesia is suboptimal and the patient is hypercarbic. Intravenous nitroglycerine is used to control hypertension below an arbitrary value of approximately 150 mmHg initially, whilst analgesia is established. Control of blood pressure with nitroglycerine reduces postoperative blood loss and lessens the risk of myocardial ischaemia due to its additional coronary vasodilator effect.

We also occasionally give sublingual nifedipine (in the absence of a suitable intravenous calcium antagonist in the UK) to control hypertension.

## Acute blood loss

The level of acceptable blood loss, as measured by chest drainage, varies depending on the extent of surgery. The blood loss during the first hour may be spuriously high as blood and fluid, which has collected during closure, empties through the drains, aided by the change from a supine to an upright sitting position. A blood loss of 2 ml/kg/hour, thereafter, is a cause for concern after a routine thoracotomy. If this bleeding continues for over 3 hours and a clotting screen is normal then re-exploration is warranted, although any clotting defect should be rectified. After an operation involving an extensive bloody surgical dissection (e.g. extrapleural pneumonectomy for a lung destroyed by chronic infection) this level of bleeding is usually tolerated over a period of 6–12 hours with appropriate transfusion of blood and clotting factors.

If blood loss persists postoperatively frequent postoperative chest X-rays are indicated to ensure that blood is not sequestrating within the chest and that blood loss is not underestimated. Significant blood clot within the pleural space is an indication for re-exploration even if visible blood losses are acceptable. A chronic haemothorax leads to an unnecessarily complicated postoperative course with frequent dysrhythmias, episodic hypotension and a potential site for infection at a later stage.

Volume requirements may also be underestimated in patients with a large amount of blood clot within the chest. Induction of anaesthesia for re-exploration and a change to the lateral position further compromises venous return and cardiac output and can result in profound hypotension. Further transfusion or even vasoconstrictor therapy may be indicated at this stage. It is essential, therefore, that the surgical team are 'scrubbed' ready to re-open the chest and remove the blood clot as soon as possible.

### Dysrhythmias

Supraventricular dysrhythmias, particularly atrial fibrillation, are common following thoracic surgery. These occur more frequently in the elderly and after pneumonectomy, particularly if there has been intra-pericardial dissection. The onset of dysrhythmias is usually delayed until 2–5 days postoperatively. We do not start prophylactic anti-dysrhythmic drugs in the pre-operative period, therefore, but wait until the extent of surgery is revealed and whether there is a significant occurrence of supraventricular dysrhythmias intra-operatively. If we feel prophylaxis is warranted we give digoxin intravenously during surgery, having checked and corrected serum potassium levels, and complete digitalization postoperatively. In this way the onset of atrial fibrillation may be prevented. At least the ventricular rate will be controlled, however, should atrial fibrillation occur.

If prophylaxis is not employed, and atrial fibrillation occurs postoperatively, then rapid intravenous digitalization can bring the heart rate under control within a few hours. Beta-adrenergic blockade is an alternative to digoxin therapy, particularly in the hypertensive patient previously receiving this medication. Verapamil also has a role in re-establishing sinus rhythm but should be used with extreme care in the hypotensive patient. Occasionally, direct current (DC) conversion is indicated to re-establish sinus rhythm promptly.

Significant ventricular dyrhythmias are treated conventionally with lignocaine or amiodarone once obvious aetiological factors such as hypoxaemia and hypokalaemia have been corrected.

## Postoperative analgesia

Adequate analgesia is essential following thoracotomy, not only in order to relieve the patient's personal distress, but also to improve lung function, allow effective physiotherapy and early mobilization and reduce the incidence of postoperative complications. The provision of adequate pain relief post-thoracotomy is a major problem, however, because of the destructive nature of the surgery and the extensive innervation of the hemithorax. Pain arises from a number of different sources. These include the chest wall and most of the pleura via the intercostal nerves, the diaphragmatic pleura via the phrenic nerves, the mediastinal pleura via the vagus nerve and the shoulder joint by way of the spinal nerves (C5–C7). The very nature of this innervation does lend itself to the use of regional techniques of anaesthesia, however, and these are in widespread use following thoracic surgery (Table 9.7).

**Table 9.7 Regional anaesthetic techniques for thoracic surgery**

---

*Intercostal nerve block*
Relatively simple to perform intra-operatively. Main disdavantages are short duration of action (unless indwelling intercostal catheters are sited) and failure to ameliorate pain from the diaphragmatic pleura, mediastinal structures and areas supplied by the posterior primary rami

*Cryoanalgesia intercostal block*
Application of extreme cold (-20 to -60°C) under direct vision to the intercostal nerves. Produces disruption of impulse transmission lasting several months. Decline in popularity due to poor analgesic results and possible association with chronic post-thoracotomy pain. Late postoperative pain is not uncommon following thoracotomy, however, and this causal relationship is not definitely established

*Intrapleural block*
Local anaesthetic agent is infused between the visceral and parietal pleura via an indwelling catheter. Analgesic action is due to widespread intercostal nerve block. This does not spread to the intercostal space. Analgesia is unpredictable due to variable loss of drug into the chest drains, binding with blood in the thorax, and rapid systemic absorption

*Paravertebral block*
Percutaneously inserted catheter at one site allows considerable spread of drug between adjacent paravertebral spaces. Provides good analgesia of both anterior and posterior primary rami. Main disadvantages are problems of accurate siting and easy displacement

*Epidural block*
Thoracic epidural block with local anaesthetic agents provides excellent analgesia but side effects with extensive sympathetic blockade limit the usefulness of this technique. Epidural block with opioids, combined with low-dose local anaesthetic agents, are now more popular by either the thoracic or lumbar route

---

The literature on pain control after thoracic surgery is vast, but this subject has been well reviewed by Kavanagh *et al.* (1994).

It is impossible to discuss every mode of analgesia in detail in a text of this nature. Preferred methods of pain relief will certainly differ from unit to unit and will depend on a number of factors. These include surgical case mix, medical and nursing expertise, seniority of medical staff, time available and level of recovery/HDU facilities. Our practice of pain relief has evolved over a number of years but is relatively simplistic, using techniques which have proven to be effective with a minimum risk to the patient. Different techniques (listed in Table 9.7) may be equally effective and safe in the hands of others. Our approach to postoperative analgesia is discussed below.

## Choice of analgesic technique

Patients scheduled for lung resection and oesophageal surgery are encouraged to accept epidural analgesia. High-risk patients are advised that this is the most suitable form of analgesia for them, unless there are specific contraindications. Those undergoing lesser procedures, such as video-assisted thoracoscopic surgery (VATS), are usually managed with intravenous opioid drugs unless their operation is likely to be particularly painful (e.g. pleurectomy). Patients who decline epidural analgesia and those in whom epidural block is contraindicated, or difficult to establish, are also managed with intravenous opioids. The group managed with intravenous opioids may also require supplementation of their analgesia with non-steroidal anti-inflammatory drugs (NSAIDs) or α-2 adrenoreceptor agonists.

## Intravenous opioids

Intravenous morphine is the major opioid we currently use postoperatively to supplement and continue the effect of either morpine or fentanyl given intra-operatively. The morphine is administered via a patient controlled analgesia (PCA) device or as a continuous infusion, at a rate controlled by the nursing staff. The effect of analgesia is monitored on a verbal scale by the nurses and noted on a chart or computer record.

In the initial phase of recovery morphine boluses of 2–4 mg are given to establish adequate analgesia. Thereafter an infusion rate of 1–5 mg of morphine per hour is usually satisfactory. In fit, relatively young patients we also add a small dose of droperidol to the morphine infusion as an anti-emetic (droperidol 2.5 mg in a solution of 30 mg morphine in 30 ml 5% dextrose).

Intravenous opioid analgesia has well known and significant side effects including respiratory depression and nausea. It is not the 'gold standard' of post-thoracotomy pain relief but is adequate in the majority of patients. If this form of pain relief is not wholly satisfactory supplementation with other drugs is indicated.

## Supplementation of intravenous opioid analgesia

Non-steroidal anti-inflammatory drugs (NSAIDs) are often very helpful in establishing good pain relief post-thoracotomy if analgesia is inadequate with intravenous opioids. We usually give diclofenac sodium (50–100mg) per rectum, although ketorolac (10–15 mg) given by intramuscular or intravenous injection is an alternative.

The combination of NSAIDs with opioids can be extremely effective but we are wary of using them routinely because of possible side effects. We have certainly seen patients drift into renal failure following the administration of NSAIDs. Exacerbation of postoperative bleeding because of their effect on platelet function is another real problem. NSAIDs are only given to patients with normal renal function and we prefer to check urea and creatinine levels, before and after surgery, if these drugs are to be used. We do not prescribe NSAIDS on a routine basis in the early postoperative period, particularly the first day, and avoid the use of NSAIDs as far as possible in the elderly. In this latter group rectal paracetamol can be helpful.

Increasing interest has been shown in the use of α-2 adrenoreceptor agonists to provide and improve postoperative analgesia by a variety of routes (Maze and Tranquill, 1991). Clonidine (2 µg/kg) can be given by slow intravenous injection to treat breakthrough pain as it seems to have a synergistic effect with morphine.

The morning after surgery oral analgesic therapy can be instituted. Co-dydramol (dihydrocodeine and paracetamol) or co-codamol (codeine phosphate and paracetamol) are usually satisfactory at this stage but NSAIDs may be more effective. NSAIDs are given orally, therefore, if pain is not adequately controlled by other means, providing there is no history of peptic ulceration and there is no renal dysfunction.

In addition to the drugs discussed above tramadol is a newer analgesic which may be useful if postoperative pain control is unsatisfactory. Tramadol produces analgesia both by an opioid effect and by enhancement of serotoninergic and adrenergic pathways. It is reported to have fewer side effects than traditional opioid drugs; in particular it is said to cause less respiratory depression.

## Epidural analgesia

Thoracic epidural analgesia with local anaesthetic agents was, at one time, considered to be the best form of analgesia following thoracotomy. A high block is required to produce satisfactory analgesia, however, and the ensuing sympathetic blockade causes a number of cardiovascular side effects. These include a decrease in cardiac output, reduction in heart rate, decreased systemic vascular resistance and a drop in mean blood pressure. These cardiovascular complications limit the usefulness of thoracic epidural analgesia with local anaesthetic agents alone and therefore increasing interest has been shown in the use of epidural opioid drugs. Epidural opioids can be administered by the thoracic or lumbar route and are often combined with a low concentration of a local anaesthetic agent. This improves the quality of analgesia without causing cardiovascular side-effects. The main complications associated with the use of epidural opioids include respiratory depression, nausea, pruritus and urinary retention.

There is now a substantial amount of literature on the use of epidural opioids for postoperative analgesia. This seems to suggest that lipophilic opioids such as fentanyl are more effective when placed in the epidural space at a level corresponding to that of the surgery (segmental effect). Conversely satisfactory analgesia can be achieved if lipophobic opioids, such as morphine, are placed in the epidural space some distance from the site of surgery. The low lipophilicity of morphine, however, means that drug present in the cerebrospinal fluid (CSF) is likely to migrate rostrally with CSF flow. This may result in delayed respiratory depression (Green, 1992).

Contrary to the discussion above we currently use diamorphine, which has a relatively high lipid solubility, via the lumbar epidural route to provide analgesia post-thoracotomy. Diamorphine has a rapid onset of action but shows a variable duration of action which may exceed morphine. This is probably due to its initial uptake into the spinal cord as diamorphine and continued action through hydrolysis to its active metabolites of mono-acetyl morphine and morphine. Diamorphine is commonly used by the epidural route in the UK but is unavailable in many other countries.

We prefer to administer epidural diamorphine via a high lumbar route and combine this with a low concentration of a local anaesthetic agent (Table 9.8). Thoracic opioid epidural analgesia may be optimal but has a number of disadvantages, which we believe outweigh the advantages. The main questions pertaining to the use of the thoracic epidural route involve its safety, ease of cannulation and whether it holds significant advantages over the lumbar route. Reports of neurological damage associated with thoracic epidurals are rare, although serious complications have occurred. The true incidence is likely to be

**Table 9.8 Epidural diamorphine – suggested regime**

---

*Site of catheter insertion*
High lumbar region ($L_1$–$L_2$ or $L_2$–$L_3$) – see text
or
Thoracic epidural block

*Initial bolus dose*
Diamorphine 1.5–2 mg made up to 20 ml in 0.1% bupivacaine
Give the 20 ml (after a test dose) before the skin incision

*Infusion*
Diamorphine 10 mg in 50 ml
Diamorphine made up to 50 ml total volume with 10 ml plain 0.5% bupivacaine plus normal saline. (i.e. 0.1% bupivacaine)

Infusion rate:
Start at 5 ml/hour approximately 1 hour into surgery (depending on weight/age/physical status of the patient)
0–10 ml/hour in initial postoperative period
After 1–3 hours usually require less than 5 ml/hour

---

Ropivacaine would be a suitable, less toxic, substitute for bupivacaine

higher than that reported in the literature due to the medico-legal implications. Thoracic epidurals can be established with the patient awake or anaesthetized. It is safer for the patient to be awake so that the sign of shooting pain from cord puncture is not obscured by general anaesthesia. Bromage (1989) has stated that thoracic epidurals should be established only in the awake patient.

It is more difficult to identify the thoracic space than the lumbar space due to the steeper angulation of the thoracic spinous processes. In addition the epidural space is shallower in the thoracic region making dural tap more likely. Failure to identify the thoracic space is also reported at a rate of 2–10% and this reflects anatomical difficulty, level of operator experience and reluctance to persevere when the likely complications are of a very serious nature.

It is perhaps not surprising, from the above discussion, that we elect to use opioid drugs combined with low-dose bupivacaine administered via the high lumbar route. This regime provides effective analgesia with minimal complications. Ropivacaine may prove to be a more suitable local anaesthetic drug to use in this situation, however, because it produces less motor block than bupivacaine and is less cardiotoxic.

## Local anaesthetic techniques

We are not particular proponents of local anaesthetic blocks for analgesia post-thoracotomy but others use a number of techniques with considerable success (Table 9.7). Local anaesthetic intercostal and paravertebral blocks can certainly be effective in reducing parenteral opioid requirements in the first few hours post-surgery and we utilize this technique in some patients. In the past we have used cryoablation of the intercostal nerves but have largely discontinued this technique because of the dysasthesia it can produce in the medium- to long-term.

## Miscellaneous management problems

### Thromboprophylaxis

Anti-thrombosis prophylaxis is employed in all patients except young 'fit' patients having short operations. Anti-thromboembolism stockings are prescribed even in this group, however.

Other patients are classified as at moderate or high risk of developing postoperative venous thromboembolism and are treated accordingly.

Moderate-risk patients are considered to be all those having major surgery together with debilitated patients having any type of operation. High-risk patients are listed in Table 9.9. Moderate- and high-risk patients are nursed with stockings and given low molecular weight heparin (Fragmin) peri-operatively on the regime shown in Table 9.10. There is evidence that low molecular weight heparins are as effective as unfractionated heparin in the prevention of venous thrombo-embolism and may be more effective in orthopaedic practice. They have a longer duration of action than unfractionated heparin and once daily subcutaneous dosage means they are convenient to use. Standard prophylactic regimes do not require monitoring and there appear to be fewer bleeding problems with the use of low molecular weight heparin. Recent opinion (Horlocker, 1998) suggests that there remains a problem relating to the use of low molecular weight heparins and the formation of epidural haematoma after catheter insertion.

### Antibiotic therapy

Antibiotic prophylaxis is controversial and should be kept simple. The majority of patients are given a cephalosporin such as cephazolin during, or just after, the

---

**Table 9.9 Patients considered to be high risk for thromboembolism**

- All patients with malignancy
- Patients with a previous history of deep vein thrombosis (DVT)
- Patients with morbid obesity
- Patients above the age of 65 years
- Patients on an oral contraceptive. This should, preferably, be stopped one month prior to surgery. HRT is continued

---

**Table 9.10 Anti-thromboembolism regime – thoracic surgery**

*Moderate risk*
Low molecular weight heparin (Fragmin) 2500 i.u. by subcutaneous injection 1–2 hours pre-operatively, then 2500 i.u. daily for 5 days

*High risk*
Low molecular weight heparin (Fragmin) 2500 i.u. by subcutaneous injection 1–2 hours pre-operatively, then 2500 i.u. 12 hours later. Maintain on 5000 i.u. daily for 5 days

All patients should continue with anti-thromboembolism stockings until such time as they are fully mobile

induction of anaesthesia and continued for 24 hours postoperatively. Antibiotic prophylaxis is particularly important if surgery is planned to involve the opening of the trachea, bronchus or oesophagus or if the patient is immunosuppressed.

Metronidazole is given in addition to cephazolin in all patients undergoing tracheal resection, oesophagectomy and excision of abdominal metastases.

Postoperatively any patient with a temperature greater than 38°C should have blood and sputum cultures taken together with any other relevant specimens for microbiology (e.g. urine, wound swabs, etc.). If a central line is in place it should be removed and replaced (if necessary) and the tip sent for culture. Empirical treatment with antibiotics is indicated if a patient is expectorating purulent sputum after pulmonary resection, particularly when febrile. A chest infection following lung resection is life-threatening and should be treated vigorously preferably following advice from the microbiologists. Choice of antibiotic will depend on local circumstances and, once available, sputum cultures.

## Renal failure

Renal failure does occur following thoracotomy and contributes to mortality. Causative factors include pre-existing renal dysfunction, dehydration, cardiovascular complications and the use of nephrotoxic drugs such as aminoglycoside antibiotics and NSAIDs.

Urinary retention is common following thoracotomy particularly in elderly male patients and those managed with epidural analgesia. If there is any doubt concerning urine output a urinary catheter should be inserted. It is important that a urine output of greater than 0.5 ml/kg/hour is maintained in the immediate postoperative period. Any patient who has not achieved this must be carefully assessed to ensure that he or she is not clinically hypovolaemic or negative in terms of overall fluid balance. Fluid overload is deleterious as far as the lungs are concerned but dehydration is detrimental to renal function. If fluid balance is thought to be satisfactory low-dose dopamine may be indicated but it is important to exclude, and treat, hypovolaemia prior to using a diuretic such as frusemide to promote urine output. In this situation a diuretic will only exacerbate hypovolaemia and renal failure.

If there is any doubt concerning the aetiology and treatment of a poor urine output expert advice should be sought from a renal physician.

## Nutrition

Patients presenting for lung resection are rarely grossly cachectic or malnourished, although they may have lost some weight. Following thoracotomy patients should be encouraged to supplement their oral diet with liquid calorie and protein supplements. Occasionally it is necessary to place a fine bore nasogastric tube to provide a route for enteral feeding. In general, however, we try and avoid the use of nasogastric tubes as they are uncomfortable to the patient and interfere with coughing and sputum clearance.

Patients with oesophageal obstruction are likely to be grossly malnourished and may need enteral feeding pre-operatively either through a fine bore nasogastric tube placed through the obstruction or via a percutaneous endoscopic gastrostomy (PEG) feeding tube. Occasionally, total parenteral nutrition (TPN) may be instituted by intravenous infusion but the enteral route is preferred.

# References

Bardoczky G.I., Levarlet M., Engelman E. and Defrancquen P. (1993) Continuous spirometry for detection of double-lumen endobrochial tube displacement. *Br J Anaesth;* **70:** 499–502.

Bromage P.R. (1989) The control of post-thoracotomy pain. *Anaesthesia;* **44:** 445–446.

Entwistle M.D., Roe P.G., Sapsford D.J. *et al.* (1991) Patterns of oxygenation after thoracotomy. *Br J Anaesth;* **67:** 704–711.

Green D.W. (1992) The clinical use of spinal opioids. In *Anaesthesia Review* (Ed. Kaufman L.). Churchill Livingstone, Edinburgh, Vol. 9, pp. 80–111.

Horlocker T.T. and Wedel D.J. (1998) Spinal and epidural blockade and perioperative low molecular weight heparin: smooth sailing on the Titanic. *Anaesth. Analg.;* **86:** 1153–1156.

Kam A.C., O'Brien M. and Kam P.C.A. (1993) Pleural drainage systems. *Anaesthesia;* **48:** 154–161.

Kavanagh B.P., Katz J. and Sandler A.N. (1994) Pain control after thoracic surgery. A review of current techniques. *Anesthesiology;* **81:** 737–759.

Maze M. and Tranquill W. (1991) Alpha-2 adrenoreceptor agonists. Defining the role in clinical anesthesia. *Anesthesiology;* **74:** 581–605.

Simon B.A., Hurford W. E., Alfille P.H. *et al.* (1992) An aid to the diagnosis of malpositioned double-lumen tubes. *Anesthesiology;* **76:** 845.

Slinger P.D. (1995) Perioperative fluid management for thoracic surgery: the puzzle of post-pneumonectomy pulmonary edema. *J Cardiothorac Vasc Anesth;* **9:** 442–451.

# Further reading

Goldstraw P. (1987) Postoperative management of the thoracic surgical patient. In *Thoracic Anaesthesia*. Clinical Anaesthesiology (Ed. Gothard J.W.W.). Baillière Tindall, London, Vol. 1, pp. 207–231.

# Appendix: Temporary cardiac pacing

Temporary cardiac pacing may be necessary following cardiac surgery; thus it is necessary for the anaesthetist to have a basic knowledge of the classification and function of the various modes of pacemaker available. It is, however, usual for a pacing technician or cardiologist to be available for advice if required.

Temporary pacemakers are currently classified using a three letter code according to the chamber paced, the chamber sensed and the pacemaker response (Table 1). Permanent pacemakers have additional codes for programmability and antitachyarrhythmic functions. The pacing wires are applied to the ventricular and/or atrial epicardium intra-operatively, and the appropriate mode selected. The indications for commonly used modes of temporary pacing are shown in Table 2.

**Table 1 Temporary pacemaker codes**

| Chamber(s) paced | Chamber(s) sensed | Response to sensing |
| --- | --- | --- |
| 0 = none | 0 = none | 0 = none |
| A = atrium | A = atrium | T = triggered |
| V = ventricle | V = ventricle | I = inhibited |
| D = dual (atrium + ventricle) | D = Dual (atrium + ventricle) | D = Dual (triggered + inhibited) |

**Table 2 Common modes of cardiac pacing used in the early postoperative period**

| Mode | Function | Indications |
| --- | --- | --- |
| VVI | Paces the ventricle Senses the ventricle Inhibits activity | Absence of organized atrial activity with intermittent AV block |
| VDD | Paces the ventricle Senses both chambers Inhibits and stimulates | Normal sinus node function with AV block |
| DDI | Paces both chambers Senses both chambers Inhibits | Sinus node dysfunction with intact AV conduction |
| DDD | Paces both chambers Senses both chambers Inhibits and stimulates | Normal sinus node function with compromised AV conduction |
| AAI | Paces the atrium Senses the atrium Inhibits the atrium | Sinus node dysfunction with normal AV conduction |
| AOO | Paces the atrium regardless of the intrinsic rhythm | The need for temporary atrial pacing in the presence of significant electromagnetic noise which may inappropriately inhibit the pacemaker |

# Index